MW00980373

# LASER HAIR REMOVAL

*This book is dedicated to my wife, Rachel, and my children, Lauren, Sarah, Brad and Tara. Without their support, love and never-ending patience, this text would have simply remained a dream and not a reality*

# LASER HAIR REMOVAL

DAVID J GOLDBERG MD
Chief of Dermatologic Surgery at New Jersey Medical School, Adjunct
Professor of Law at Fordham University School of Law, Skin Laser and
Surgery Specialists of New York and New Jersey, and Director, Skin
Laser Center, Pascack Valley Hospital, Westwood, NJ, USA

With contributions from Robert N Richards MD
and Steven Mulholland MD

Martin Dunitz

© 2000 Martin Dunitz Ltd, a member of the Taylor & Francis group

First published in the United Kingdom in 2000
by Martin Dunitz Ltd, The Livery House, 7–9 Pratt Street, London NW1 0AE

Tel:      +44 (0) 20 7482 2202
Fax:      +44 (0) 20 7267 0159
E-mail:   info.dunitz@tandf.co.uk
Website:  http:/ / www.dunitz.co.uk

**Reprinted 2002**

All rights reserved. No part of this publication may be reproduced, stored in a retrieval system, or transmitted, in any form or by any means, electronic, mechanical, photocopying, recording, or otherwise, without the prior permission of the publisher or in accordance with the provisions of the Copyright, Designs and Patents Act 1988 or under the terms of any licence permitting limited copying issued by the Copyright Licensing Agency, 90 Tottenham Court Road, London W1P 0LP.

Although every effort has been made to ensure that drug doses and other information are presented accurately in this publication, the ultimate responsibility rests with the prescribing physician. Neither the publishers nor the authors can be held responsible for errors or for any consequences arising from the use of information contained herein. For detailed prescribing information or instructions on the use of any product or procedure discussed herein, please consult the prescribing information or instructional material issued by the manufacturer.

A CIP record for this book is available from the British Library.

ISBN 1 85317 831 4

Distributed in the USA by
Fulfilment Center
Taylor & Francis
7625 Empire Drive
Florence, KY 41042, USA
Toll Free Tel.: +1 800 634 7064
E-mail: cserve@routledge_ny.com

Distributed in the rest of the world by
Thomson Publishing Services Cheriton House
North Way, Andover
Hampshire SP10 5BE, UK
Tel.: +44 (0) 1264 332424
E-mail:
salesorder.tandf@thomsonpublishingservices.co.uk

Distributed in Canada by
Taylor & Francis
74 Rolark Drive
Scarborough, Ontario M1R 4G2, Canada
Toll Free Tel.: +1 877 226 2237
E-mail: tal_fran@istar.ca

Composition by 𝍏 Tek-Art, Croydon, Surrey

Printed and bound in Singapore by Kyodo Printing Co (S'pore) Pte Ltd

# CONTENTS

# PREFACE

Humans, for the most part, consider hair for its cosmetic significance. Patients seeking treatment of excess or, more commonly, unwanted hair present with a variety of psychosocial complaints. Only rarely do individuals seek non-cosmetic hair removal.

Lasers and light sources are successfully used to treat a variety of vascular and pigmented lesions. Only over the last few years has there been interest in the role of these technologies in the treatment of unwanted hair. This book explores the currently reviewed lasers and light sources available for hair removal. The first chapter of the book begins with a discussion of hair biology. A subsequent chapter reviews laser physics and its application to hair removal. Subsequent chapters evaluate both the uses of electrolysis and available laser/light sources for hair removal. Each chapter reviews research studies, currently available technologies, and discusses the author's approach to using each system. Finally, a chapter is dedicated to the business aspects of a hair removal practice.

# ACKNOWLEDGMENTS

The author and publishers would like to thank Robert N Richards, MD, FRCP(C), of Toronto, Canada, who kindly contributed the text and illustrations for Chapter 3, and Steven Mulholland, MD, of Toronto, Canada, who kindly contributed Chapter 10.

The author and publishers would also like to thank M Grossman, MD, for the kind loan of Figures 6.5, 6.37, 6.38, and 6.42.

# 1 HAIR BIOLOGY

## KEY POINTS

(1) Growth in hair follicles is cyclical and has three stages: anagen (growing phase), telogen (resting phase), and catagen (regression phase)

(2) The exact identity of all the components of the growth center(s) of hair is controversial

(3) Hair growth centers lie deep in the dermis, so the energy required to remove hair is significant and has to be balanced against the risk of damage to the epidermis

(4) People seek hair removal treatment not only for cosmetic reasons but also because of hypertrichosis or hirsutism resulting from disease or medication

## ANATOMY

Hair follicles develop embryologically through a complex series of interactions between the epidermis and dermis. Hair follicles, anatomically, consist of three distinct units: the hair bulb, isthmus, and infundibulum. The hair bulb, one of three pluripotential hair growth sites, is the region that extends from the base of the follicle to the insertion site of the arrector pili muscle. The isthmus and infundibulum are not thought to play any role in hair growth. The other two sites of pluripotential hair cells are thought to be the 'bulge' at the site of the arrector pili muscle insertion and the dermal papilla (Figure 1.1).

The bulbar region of the hair follicle contains a pool of relatively undifferentiated epithelial cells, termed matrix cells, which give rise to the hair and its surrounding inner root sheath. During the growing phase (*anagen*) of the hair cycle, these matrix cells proliferate extremely rapidly. After a period of active growth in anagen, matrix cells cease to divide, and the lower follicle regresses during catagen. When the regression is completed, the follicle enters *telogen*, a resting phase that lasts for several

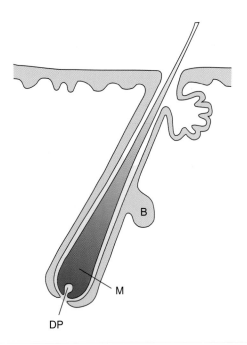

**Figure 1.1.** Hair follicle with dermal papilla (DP), matrix (M) and bulge (B)

B

M

DP

months. The matrix cells then resume proliferation and produce a new hair bulb, thus re-entering anagen and completing the hair cycle.[1,2]

It has generally been assumed that matrix cells, through their interactions with the dermal papilla, play the pivotal central role in follicular growth and differentiation. However, research evaluating growth of new hair has revealed that the matrix is not the only growth center.

Although the dermal papilla is not technically part of the actual hair, it remains a very important site for future hair induction. It is also the major probable site of melanin production in terminal hairs. It is this melanin that absorbs visible light and lasers used to remove unwanted pigmented hair. Hair follicle stem cells reside not only within the hair bulb matrix and dermal papilla, but also in the pluripotential hair-forming cells in the bulge, a component of hair outer root sheath cells located in the mid-portion of the follicle at the arrector pili muscle attachment site (Figure 1.1). All of these sites can induce new hair formation.

All human hairs show various stages of hair growth.[3] The anagen, or growth phase, leads to the catagen or regression phase. The telogen or resting phase follows, just prior to the resumption of the anagen phase. The anagen growth phase is variable in duration and can last up to 6 years depending on the site. The relatively constant catagen phase is generally of 3 weeks' duration, whereas the telogen phase usually lasts approximately 3 months (Figures 1.2 and 1.3). At any given time, the majority of the hair follicles (80–85%) are in anagen and the remaining follicles are either in the catagen phase (2%) or the telogen phase (10–15%). However, anagen and telogen phases do vary from anatomic site to site (Table 1.1).

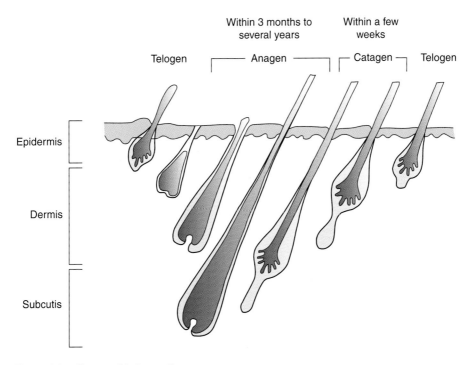

Epidermis

Dermis

Subcutis

Telogen — Anagen — Catagen — Telogen

Within 3 months to several years

Within a few weeks

**Figure 1.2.** Stages of hair growth

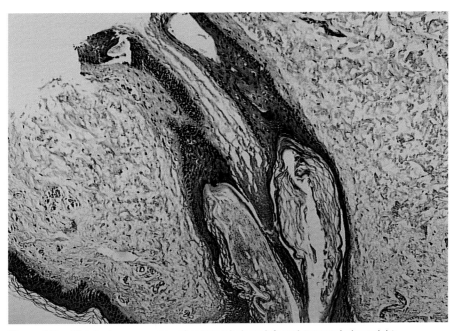

**Figure 1.3.** Histologic appearance of catagen hair on left and anagen hair on right

3

| Body area | Duration (months) | | % Telogen |
| | Anagen | Telogen | |
|---|---|---|---|
| Scalp | 48–72 | 3–4 | 10–15 |
| Eyelashes | 1.0–1.5 | – | – |
| Eyebrows | 1–2 | 3–4 | 85–94 |
| Moustache | 2–5 | 1.5 | 34 |
| Beard | 12 | 2.5 | – |
| Chest | – | 2.5 | – |
| Axillae | – | – | 31–79 |
| Arms | 1–3 | 2–4 | 72–86 |
| Thighs | 1–2 | 2–3 | 64–83 |
| Legs | 4–6 | 3–6 | 62–88 |
| Pubic | – | – | 65–81 |

**Table 1.1.** Human hair cycles (derived from Olsen[19])

# GROWTH CENTERS OF HAIR

Long-term hair removal requires that a laser or light source impact on one or more growth centers of hair. In order to do so, an appropriate target or chromophore must be identified. The major growth center has always been thought to be the hair matrix. However, as described above, new hairs may evolve from the dermal papilla, follicular matrix or the 'bulge'.

It is the bulbar region of the hair follicle that contains the matrix cells; a pool of relatively undifferentiated epithelial cells. These have been thought to give rise to the hair and its surrounding inner root sheath. During the growing anagen phase of the hair cycle, these matrix cells proliferate extremely rapidly with a doubling time of 18–24 hours. This proliferation appears to be tightly controlled. Not only does it depend on adjacent population of specialized mesenchymal cells, which form the dermal papilla, but it is also cyclic. After this period of active growth in anagen, matrix cells cease to divide, and the lower follicle regresses during catagen. When the regression is completed, the follicle enters telogen. The matrix cells then resume proliferation and produce a new hair bulb, thus re-entering anagen and completing a hair cycle.

Although it has generally been assumed that matrix cells, through their interactions with the dermal papilla, play a central role in follicular growth and differentiation, it has been noted that a complete hair follicle can be regenerated after the matrix-containing hair follicle is surgically removed. In addition, the controlling mechanism responsible for the cyclic growth of the hair has been enigmatic.

Earlier theories on recapitulation of the anagen cycle focused on the necessary preservation of the hair matrix (the putative site of follicular stem cells) and the contiguous dermal papillae.[4] However, we now know from the elegant transection experiments of Oliver[5,6] on rat vibrissae, that if the dermal papilla and not more than the lower one-third of the follicle is removed, the hair follicle can regenerate. Oliver also found that when lengths of the lower third of the vibrissae follicle wall, but not lengths of the upper two-thirds of the follicle wall, were transplanted into ear skin, whiskers were again produced.[7] From these experiments, it was clearly established that the outer root sheath and the adherent mesenchymal layer from the lower follicle were, in the absence of a matrix and dermal papilla, the essential elements in the regeneration of the hair follicle. Additional studies then addressed the issue of whether it was the outer root sheath cells in the upper third of the follicle that were incapable of supporting whisker growth or of stimulating papilla formation, or whether the mesenchymal cells at this level were incompetent to form a dermal papilla.[8] Oliver evaluated the removal of different lengths of follicle so that less than or equal to half of the upper region of the follicle was left in situ. After the cut whisker shafts were plucked from these follicle remnants, the mouths of the follicular tubes left by the plucked whisker were left open, or isolated dermal papillae were placed there. Fourteen of 19 of the follicular segments with papilla implants produced whisker's versus none of the follicular segments without papilla implants. This confirmed that non-regeneration of papillae and whiskers from the upper two-thirds of the follicle arose from the inability of the mesenchymal layer to form papillae at this level and not from the incompetence of the outer root sheath to become organized for hair production. Another study by Oliver[9] examined hair regeneration from the standpoint of papilla preservation as opposed to full follicle requirement. He found that isolated vibrissae papillae could induce follicle formation from ear epidermis.

Although the dermal papilla is clearly critical to growth, it can be replaced by mesodermal tissue under follicular epithelial cell influence. Where and what these multipotential epithelium-derived cells may be has recently been a subject of great interest. Cotsarelis et al.[4] have determined that, in rodents at least, a group of specialized slow-cycling cells of the outer root sheath, residing in the bulge region in a fixed protected position, have properties consistent with the follicular stem cells. Whether these data can be completely reconciled with Oliver's experiments is unclear.[10] Reynolds et al.[11,12] have identified a population of germinative epidermal cells in the lower end bulb region of anagen hair follicles in both rats and humans that are distinct from epidermal or outer root sheath cells. The cells remain quiescent in culture unless cultured in association with hair follicle dermal papilla cells. In this situation, they become proliferative, aggregate, and form organotypic structures. At telogen it is not clear whether these germinative cells remain as a permanent population or are replaced or augmented by outer root sheath cells,[13] perhaps from the bulge region.

Kim and Choi[14] have recently reported human hair transection experiments, with results similar to those of Oliver. They reimplanted transected human occipital scalp hairs into non-scalp (forehead or leg) skin. Sectioning was done (1) just below the sebaceous gland (upper one-third of the follicle), (2) through the isthmus in the middle of the follicle, or (3) below the level of insertion of the arrector pili muscle bulge region (lower one-third of the follicle). Follicular transplants from the lower two-thirds, lower half and upper two-thirds of the follicle developed into normal sized hairs. Transplants from the upper one-third and lower one-third of the follicle did not regenerate hair. Follicular transplants from the upper half of the follicle produced fine hairs. They concluded that the mid-follicle or isthmus portion of the follicle is necessary for regeneration of the hair follicle.

In terms of permanent hair removal, the aforementioned data are extremely important. Such data shift the potential target of destruction, from the hair matrix and dermal papilla alone, to other more superficial areas of the hair follicle as well.

# 'Stem Cells'

A key issue that must be addressed when one considers the homeostasis and differentiation of any self-renewing tissue such as the hair follicle is the location of the 'stem cells'. Based on studies of stem cells of the hemopoietic system and various epithelial systems, we know that stem cells possess many of the following properties:

(1)  they are relatively undifferentiated both ultrastructurally and biochemically,
(2)  they have a large proliferative potential and are responsible for the long-term maintenance and regeneration of the tissue,
(3)  they are normally slow cycling, presumably to conserve their proliferative potential and to minimize DNA errors that could occur during replication,
(4)  they can be stimulated to proliferate in response to wounding and certain growth stimuli,
(5)  they are often located in close proximity to a population of rapidly proliferating cells and
(6)  they are usually found in a well-protected, highly vascularized and innervated area.

Such a discrete population of primitive stem cells has been definitely identified in mouse hair follicles and is probably present in human follicles as well. These cells are slow cycling, possess a relatively undifferentiated cytoplasm, and are well protected (they always remain intact and are left behind after hair plucking). Surprisingly, the location of these cells is not the matrix area of the bulb – the location of known follicular stem cells. Instead, such cells appear to be located in a specific area of the outer root sheath called the 'Wulst' or bulge. This is, as described above, at the attachment site of the arrector pili muscle. It is below the opening of the sebaceous gland and marks the lower end of the 'permanent' portion of the hair follicle.

Keratinocytes below it degenerate during catagen and telogen phases of the hair cycle. In embryonic hair, the bulge is a prominent structure, sometimes even larger than the hair bulb. It remains fairly inconspicuous in routine paraffin sections of adult human and animal follicles.[4]

Although evidence clearly suggests several potential growth centers in hair, there are several biological advantages for the location of follicular stem cells to be in the bulge area instead of the lower bulb. First, unlike the hair bulb, which undergoes cyclic degeneration, cells in the bulge area are in the permanent portion of the hair follicle. Situated at the lower end of the permanent portion, bulge cells are in a strategically convenient position to interact, during late telogen, with the upcoming papilla and to send out a new follicular downgrowth during early anagen. Second, basal cells of the bulge form an outgrowth pointing away from the hair shaft and are therefore safeguarded against accidental loss due to plucking. The bulb area, conversely, is vulnerable to damage from plucking. Finally, the bulge area is a reasonably well-vascularized area so that cells in this area are well nourished.

# MECHANISMS OF CESSATION/REACTIVATION OF GROWTH

Although the histologic changes occurring during the growing anagen, regressing catagen, and resting telogen phases of the hair cycle are more-or-less clear, the mechanistic basis underlying the cessation and reactivation of the follicular growth has remained obscure. The recognition that hair follicle stem cells may reside in the bulge area would help to explain the critical events during the various phases of the human hair cycle. In such a model, during late telogen or early anagen, dermal papilla cells activate the normally slow-cycling stem cells of the bulge area. The mechanism of this activation is unknown, but could involve a diffusible dermal papilla-derived growth factor and/or direct cell–cell contact. Such a sequence is known to occur during a comparable stage in embryonic hair formation. This activation would then lead to proliferation of the germinal cells of the bulge area, which forms a downgrowth. As the dermal papilla is pushed away from the bulge by this newly formed epithelial column, the bulge stem cells presumably return to their normally quiescent, slow-cycling stage in mid-anagen.

The dermal papilla is known to undergo hair cycle-dependent changes in its volume, histologic appearance, and basement membrane composition. During most phases of the hair cycle, the dermal papilla appears to be relatively dormant. However, during mid-anagen, there is a burst of cell proliferation in the dermal papilla. Some of these replicating papillary cells are endothelial cells engaged in angiogenesis, which occurs in the perifollicular area. Possible consequences of this activation include the formation of new blood vessels that would undoubtedly facilitate rapid hair growth.

Since almost 100% of matrix cells are involved in continuous replication, they are probably derived from the putative stem cells that reside in the distant bulge area. According to this concept, stem cells can potentially live the entire life of a human being and are slow cycling. After each stem cell division, on average one of the two (probably identical) daughter cells leaves the stem cell 'home' – the bulge. Such cells ultimately become matrix cells. Such matrix cells, by definition, have only a limited prolaterative potential. They eventually become exhausted and undergo terminal differentiation – a new hair is born. The length of the anagen phase that now starts is an intrinsic trait of its beginning matrix cell. This may explain why, once started, the length of the growing phase is relatively insensitive to environmental factors. This anagen phase is then followed by catagen. During early catagen, the dermal papilla is condensed and becomes increasingly distant from the regressing matrix. They are still connected, however, by an epithelial sheath. Later, the dermal papilla is pulled upward, presumably through the contractile activities of the outer root sheath cells and/or the connective sheath cells that wrap around the dermal papilla. This upward movement of the dermal papilla apparently plays a critical role in the subsequent activation of cells in the bulge area.

Anecdotal approaches have suggested that the pluripotential cells of the bulge, dermal papilla, and hair matrix must be treated in the anagen cycle for effective hair removal. If the damage is not permanent during this cycle, it has been suggested, follicles will move into the telogen stage as they fall out. Thus, all of the follicles may become synchronized after the first laser treatment. The hair follicle will then return to anagen, according to the natural hair cycle. This cycle varies depending on the anatomic location. It is shortest on the face and longer on the body.

# THE HAIR GROWTH CYCLE AND ITS IMPLICATIONS

Despite variations in length, growing phases, and type of hair, all human hair growth is cyclical. It is during the anagen growth phase that the hair bulb encases the dermal papillae. In the lowest regions of the hair bulb, melanocytes actively transfer melanin to the dividing matrix cells. With time, the matrix cells move more superficially in the hair bulb. With this movement, they begin to differentiate into portions of the hair shaft, as well as inner and outer root sheaths. It is the outer root sheath that anchors a hair in place. At the end of this anagen growing stage, deeper matrix keratinocytes cease proliferation and undergo terminal differentiation. It is this process that results in involution of the lower follicle. The melanization of hair ceases just before the conclusion of anagen. At this time, the follicular bulb begins to move more superficially in the dermis. The connective tissue sheath that surrounds the entire hair shaft and outer root sheath begins to terminally differentiate at the level of the isthmus – an area between the sebaceous duct and the arrector pili muscle insertion. This process leads to a tenuous hold of the telogen hair to the follicle. Thus, during telogen, it is easier to pull hairs from their 'roots'. After a period that appears fairly fixed for most anatomic areas, the hair is shed and a new anagen cycle begins.

The mouse hair follicle shows similarities and differences when compared with the human hair follicle. In the mouse hair follicle, the hair growth cycle is a continuous process; definition of clearly defined follicular growth stages (as in humans) becomes arbitrary. It was Dry[15] who first divided the cycle into three stages: anagen, the period of activity; catagen, the period of regression; and telogen, the period of quiescence. Chase[16] further divided the mouse anagen stage into six substages (I–VI). The studied mice were born with neither hair nor pigment in their skin; as the hair follicle buds enter anagen (days 1–17 of the cycle), melanin is produced and incorporated into the budding matrix.

During the first 3 days (anagen I–II) of the anagen stage, in this animal model, no melanin production is apparent and the skin remains pink. At this time, the base of the follicle is characteristically about 250µm below the skin surface and at a quiescent level. In anagen II (days 3–4 of the cycle), the follicle attains its maximum depth of at least 500µm below the skin surface. The hair usually goes no deeper.[17] Melanocytes appear along the papilla cavity, producing and transferring melanin granules to cells in the matrix, and the skin starts to turn gray. By anagen V (day 8 of the cycle), the tip of the hair has broken through the tip of the internal sheath and has grown to about the level of the epidermis. The activity of melanogenesis reaches a peak on days 8–12 (anagen V–VI). Now the skin appears black. Thereafter, the skin begins to turn pink as melanogenesis decreases, whereas the depth of the hair follicle remains at its maximum. In both the mouse and human anagen stages, the hair shaft is fully pigmented for its entire length. This would explain the finding that laser thermal damage, by way of melanin absorption, has been noted along the entire length of an anagen follicle.

When active growth ends, dramatic changes occur in the hair follicle throughout catagen.[18] Catagen is a relatively brief transitional stage (days 18–19 of the mouse cycle). Melanin production and hair growth cease abruptly. The hair shaft, in the animal model, is entirely depigmented. Since most laser systems employ melanin as the major absorbing chromophore, selective laser thermal damage along the *entire* length of catagen or telogen follicles would not be expected during these stages. During these stages, the lower hair follicle undergoes apoptosis and its base moves gradually upward to the resting position. As the hair follicle moves into telogen (days 20–24 of the cycle), hair growth and melanin production remain completely absent; stem cells remain largely quiescent.

Anagen duration varies greatly depending on age, season, anatomic region, sex, hormonal levels, and certain genetic predisposition. It is these variations that lead to the tremendous disparity in hair cycles reported by various investigators[3–5] (Table 1.1). Examples of the variations are as follows:

(1) In scalp hair there is a decrease in anagen duration with age; there is also a corresponding prolongation of the interval between loss of the telogen hair and new anagen hair regrowth.
(2) There are seasonal changes in the percentage of anagen human scalp hairs.
(3) Men show a 54-day anagen hair cycle on their thighs; women have only a 22-day cycle.
(4) Male and female anagen scalp cycles are about the same.

Although reports of anagen duration, telogen duration and percentage of hairs in telogen represent an inexact science, it is clear that when one discusses the results following laser hair removal, one must take into account the different anatomic areas in terms of anagen and telogen cycles. Since all laser and light source systems can induce temporary hair removal, only a knowledge of the anagen/telogen cycle for a particular anatomic site will determine whether this technology can induce long-term changes in the growth of hair.[19]

Thus, whether hairs are in anagen or telogen is not only of academic interest. It has been traditionally thought that it is only anagen hairs that are especially sensitive to a wide variety of destructive processes – including laser and light source damage. It is this assault on the anagen hair that leads to a metabolic disturbance of the mitotically active anagen matrix cells. The response pattern is dependent both on the duration and intensity of the insult. Three patterns of damage have been noted:

(1) premature anagen termination with subsequent start of telogen;
(2) transition from a normal to dystrophic anagen and
(3) acute matrix degeneration.

It should be noted that these changes, although well documented after a variety of physical and chemical insults, have not been well defined after laser treatment.

# LASER ENERGY REQUIRED FOR HAIR REMOVAL

Because of the depth of the hair growth centers, significant laser energies must be applied for effective hair removal. However, not only must each follicle be damaged, but also the surrounding tissue, especially the epidermis, must be protected from damage. This is required to reduce the chances of scarring and permanent pigmentary changes. Melanin, the only endogenous chromophore in the hair follicle of pigmented hair, can be effectively targeted by lasers and light sources throughout the visible light spectrum. Of the wavelengths used in currently available hair removal lasers and light sources, only the longer wavelengths are effective in destroying hair because of their greater depth of penetration. Alternatively, an exogenous chromophore, such as carbon, can be applied to the skin. This chromophore will then be irradiated with laser energy of a wavelength that matches its absorption peak. Both of the aforementioned approaches have been shown to remove hair.

# 'PERMANENCE' OF HAIR REMOVAL

Based on our current understanding of hair biology, knowledge of the hair cycle – and especially the length of telogen – becomes essential for determining whether laser or light source treatment of unwanted hair is 'temporary' or 'permanent'. Currently, there is no agreement on a definition of treatment-induced permanent hair loss. Permanence, defined as an absolute lack of hair in a treated area for the lifetime of the patient, may be an unrealistic goal.

Dierickx et al.[20] have suggested a more practical approach. They would define 'permanent' hair loss as a significant reduction in the number of terminal hairs, after a given treatment, that is stable for a period longer than the complete growth cycle of hair follicles at any given body site. Telogen may last 3–7 months on the inner thighs and chest. After telogen, the follicle will then recycle into anagen. This will also last 3–7 months. Thus hair may be considered permanently removed from these locations if there is no recurrence after this complete time period.

Olsen has suggested an even longer time period. She suggests that permanent hair reduction would be deemed to have occurred after the lapse of 6 months after one complete growth cycle.[19] If no hair regrows after this time period, it can be assumed that the growth centers have no capacity to recover from injury.

The timing of laser treatment of unwanted hair may be crucial. Selective photothermolysis requires absorption of a chromophore, such as melanin, by light. The bulb of a telogen hair is unpigmented because of the cessation of melanin production during the catagen stage. On the other hand, as anagen progresses, the bulb and papilla descend deeply into the dermis so that late anagen hairs may also be somewhat laser resistant to treatment. It would seem, therefore, that it is in early anagen that hair follicles are most sensitive to laser induced injury. Since an injury, even a laser injury, may induce telogen, the timing of a second laser treatment after the first laser-induced telogen formation, becomes critical. As the laser-resistant terminal follicles now enter an anagen growth phase, after a first treatment, the second treatment may be more effective than the first. Conversely, a second treatment given too early or too late would be expected to have little effect.

This time-honoured theory of optimal anagen treatment times has recently been challenged by Dierickx et al.[21] They evaluated 100 subjects treated with 3ms 694nm ruby laser and 5–20ms 800nm diode laser. They noted that 9 months after one treatment with either laser, 50% of the hairs lost were in anagen at the time of treatment, while 45% of the hairs lost were in telogen at the time of the initial treatment. These findings, if confirmed, would suggest that anagen/telogen cycling does not have the significant impact on laser-induced response that was previously thought.

It should be noted that there is a general consensus that hair removal results will always be effected by chosen anatomic site. Most investigators note a better response on the chest, face, legs, and axilla. Lesser responses appear to occur on the back, upper lip, and scalp. In addition, terminal hairs, and not vellus hairs respond to laser treatment. This has been shown following ruby laser treatment, but presumably applies to other lasers and light sources as well. Sacpac staining is a marker for the growth phases of hair as well as shaft damage. When Sacpac staining is undertaken, damage following laser treatment is only seen in terminal hairs. P53 staining is used as a marker of cell death. When such markers are used to evaluate hair death after laser treatment, it is the hair's external root sheath that suffers the initial damage. This damage is associated with a 5–10°C rise in follicular temperature. This has been shown to be a high enough temperature rise to cause protein denaturation, with associated hair destruction.[22]

It is now widely accepted that almost any laser can induce temporary hair loss. Fluences as low as 5J/cm² can induce this effect. The effect tends to last 1–3 months. The mechanism of action appears to be an induction of catagen and telogen. Permanent hair reduction, occurring at higher fluences, may be seen in 80% of individuals and is fluence dependent. Thus, the greater the delivered fluence, all else being equal, the better are the expected results (C Dierickx, personal communication).

# HYPERTRICHOSIS AND HIRSUTISM

An understanding of hair biology leads to improved results when unwanted hair is treated with a laser. Many individuals seeking laser hair removal are in good health. However, alterations in human biology may lead other individuals to seek laser hair removal. The development of localized or diffuse unwanted excess hair may occur in association with many inherited syndromes, as well as with the use of certain medications (especially androgens), or the presence of ovarian or adrenal tumors. Excess hair may also be seen as a normal genetic variant (Table 1.2). The use of proper terminology is confusing, yet important, in describing excess hair growth. *Hypertrichosis* is the presence of increased hair in men and women at any body site. *Hirsutism* is defined as the presence of excess hair in women only at androgen-dependent sites.[7,23,24] Hirsutism is most commonly seen on the upper chin, chest, inner thighs, back, and abdomen.

## Hirsutism

Hirsutism is caused by diseases of androgen excess or by the intake of certain medications. The most common causes are polycystic ovary syndrome (PCOS;

Virilizing tumors
    Adrenal gland
    Ovary

Endocrine disorders
    Cushing's disease

Medications
    Androgens
    Birth control pills
    Minoxidil
    Phenytoin
    Penicillamine
    Diazoxide
    Cyclosporine
    Corticosteroids
    Phenothiazines
    Haloperidol

Syndrome
    Polycystic ovary
    Malnutrition
    Porphyria
    Anorexia nervosa
    Hypothyroidism
    Dermatomyositis

**Table 1.2.** Causes of hirsutism and hypertrichosis

Stein–Leventhal syndrome) and idiopathic hirsutism. The diseases of androgen excess are usually pituitary/adrenal or ovarian in source. Elevated levels of adrenocorticotropic hormone (ACTH), which increase the adrenal secretion of cortisol, aldosterone and androgens, are a rare cause of hirsutism. Adrenal causes of hirsutism include virilizing types of congenital adrenal hyperplasia and adrenal neoplasms. Undoubtedly, PCOS is the most common cause of a disease-defined hirsutism. In the United States, 70% of patients who have PCOS show hirsutism. The severity of the androgen effect ranges from mild hirsutism to virilization. Hirsutism may also be caused by androgen-producing ovarian neoplasms. Since insulin stimulates ovarian androgen production, another ovarian cause of hirsutism is insulin resistance with its resultant hyperinsulinism.

Idiopathic hirsutism is a diagnosis of exclusion. Total testosterone levels in idiopathic hirsutisim may be normal, though free testosterone levels are high. Of note is the fact that emotional stress may cause idiopathic hirsutism.

# Hypertrichosis

Anorexia nervosa and hypothyroidism may cause hypertrichosis. Patients with anorexia nervosa frequently develop fine, dark hair growth on the face, trunk, and arms, which at times is extensive. In hypothyroidism, the hair growth is of the long, fine, soft unpigmented (vellus) type.

Although multiple drugs may cause hypertrichosis, the pathophysiology of drug-induced hypertrichosis is unknown.

# Racial Differences

All races have similar androgen and estrogen levels, despite the striking differences in amounts of body hair. Whites have more hair than do Blacks, Asians, and Native Americans. The number of hair follicles per unit of skin varies among the ethnic groups (Mediterranean > Nordic > Asian). Asians rarely have facial hair or body hair outside the pubic and axillary regions. White women of Mediterranean background have heavier hair growth and a higher incidence of excess facial hair than do those of Nordic ancestry (blond, fair-skinned). Thus, a wide range of normal hair growth exists for men and women, largely based on racial and ethnic predisposition.

# Evaluation of the Hirsute Woman

Although the overwhelming majority of patients seeking laser and light source hair removal are perfectly healthy, or present with idiopathic hirsutism, a clinical history must be undertaken to rule out those serious diseases that cause hirsutism. Histories that suggest a potential serious underlying disease include:

(1)  the onset of hirsutism that is not peripubertal;
(2)  abrupt onset and/or rapid progression of hair growth;
(3)  virilization with associated acne, male-pattern baldness, deepening of voice, increased muscle mass, decreased breast size, amenorrhea, clitoromegaly, or increased sexual drive.

If such a history is provided, a full medical evaluation is mandatory.

A careful drug history is also very important. Simple changes in drug regimens may be all that is necessary to reverse unwanted new-onset hair growth.

It can be seen, then, that although the patient's cosmetic feelings about unwanted hair growth must be considered, the physician must always be alert to rule out all the

Treatment of any underlying disease found

Suppression of androgen overproduction
    Oral contraceptives
    Dexamethasone

Blocking the effect of androgens
    Spironolactone
    Flutamide
    Cyproterone
    Finasteride

Cosmetic measures
    Shaving
    Bleaching with hydrogen peroxide
    Chemical depilatories
    Plucking
    Waxing
    Electrolysis

Weight loss

**Table 1.3.** Management options for patients with hirsutism

possible medical causes of excess hair growth.

Prior to the advent of laser and light source technology, treatment options for hair excess included treatment of associated diseases, suppression or blocking of androgen production and effect, and a variety of frustrating and/or protracted cosmetic measures (Table 1.3).

# REFERENCES

1 Abell E. Embryology and anatomy of the hair follicle. In: Olsen EA, editor. Disorders of hair growth: diagnosis and treatment. New York: McGraw-Hill;1994:1–19.
2 Conitois M, Loussouarn G, Hourseau C, Grollier JE. Ageing and hair cycles. Br J Dermatol 1995;132:86–93.
3 Seago SV, Ebling FIG. The hair cycle on the human thigh and upper arm. Br J Dermatol 1985;113:9–16.
4 Cotsarelis G, Sun TT, Lavker RM. Label-retaining cells reside in the bulge area of pilosebaceous unit: implications for follicular stem cells, hair cycle and skin carcinogenesis. Cell 1990; 61:1321–7.
5 Oliver RF. Whisker growth after removal of the dermal papilla and lengths of follicle in the hooded rat. J Embryol Exp Morphol 1966;15:331–47.

6    Oliver RF. Histological studies of whisker regeneration in the hooded rat. J Embryol Exp Morphol 1966;16:231–44.

7    Oliver RE. Ectopic regeneration of whiskers in the hooded rat from implanted lengths of vibrissa follicle wall. J Embryol Exp Morphol 1967; 17:27–34.

8    Oliver RF. The experimental induction of whisker growth in the hooded rat by implantation of dermal papillae. J Embryol Exp Morphol 1967;18:43–51.

9    Oliver RE. The induction of hair follicle formation in the adult hooded rat by vibrissa dermal papillae. J Embryol Exp Morphol 1970; 23:219–36

10   Holecek BU, Ackerman AB. Bulge-activation hypothesis: is it valid? Am J Dermatol 1993;15:235–47.

11   Reynolds AJ, Jahoda CA. Hair follicle stem cells? A distinct germinative epidermal cell population is activated in vitro by the presence of hair dermal papilla cells J Cell Sci 1991;99:373–85.

12   Reynolds AJ, Lawrence CM, Jahoda CAB. Human hair follicle germinative epidermal cell culture. J Invest Dermatol 1993;101:634S–638S.

13   Reynolds AJ, Jahoda CA. Inductive properties of hair follicle cells. Ann NY Acad Sci 1991; 642:226–41.

14   Kim JC, Choi YC. Hair follicle regeneration after horizontal resectioning: implications for hair transplantation. In: Stough DB, Haber RS, editors. Hair replacement: surgical and medical. St Louis: Mosby-Year Book;1995:355–63.

15   Dry FW. The coat of the mouse. J Genet 1926;16:287–340.

16   Chase HB. Growth of hair. Physiol Rev 1954; 34:113–26.

17   Chase HB, Rauch H, Smith VW. Critical stages of hair development and pigmentation in the mouse. Physiol Zool 1951; 24:1–8.

18   Straile WE, Chase HB, Arsenault C. Growth and differentiation of hair follicles between periods of activity and quiescence. J Exp Zool 1961;148:206–16.

19   Olsen EA. Methods of hair removal. J Am Acad Dermatol 1999; 40:143–55.

20   Dierickx CC, Grossman MC, Farinelli WA, et al. Permanent hair removal by normal mode ruby laser. Arch Dermatol 1998; 134:837–52.

21   Dierickx C, Campos VB, Lin WF, Anderson RR. Influence of hair growth cycle on efficacy of laser hair removal. Lasers Surg Med 1999; 24(suppl 11):21.

22   Topping A. Ruby laser hair destruction. Presented at Second Annual European Society for Lasers in Aesthetic Surgery, Oxford, England, March 1999.

23   Wheeland RG. Laser-assisted hair removal. Dermatol Clin 1997; 15:469–77.

24   Goldberg DJ. Unwanted hair: evaluation and treatment with lasers and light source technology. Adv Dermatol 1999; 14:115–39.

# 2 LASER PHYSICS

## KEY POINTS

(1) 'Laser' is an acronym for light amplification by the stimulated emission of radiation
(2) Laser light is monochromatic (one wavelength), coherent (in phase), and collimated (parallel light waves)
(3) Laser light is absorbed by melanin chromophores – in the skin and hair – and converted into heat which can be exploited to destroy hair
(4) The impact of laser light on hair and skin varies with energy fluence, wavelength, pulse width, and spot size

## DEFINITIONS

Light, whether emitted from a laser or light source, is a complex system of radiant energy composed of waves and energy bundles (photons) that are ordered in the electromagnetic spectrum according to the size of the waves. This *wavelength*, or distance between two successive wave crests, determines the color of visible light. Additionally each source of electromagnetic energy has a given *frequency*, which is the number of waves passing a point per second.

The word *laser* is an acronym for light amplification by the stimulated emission of radiation. The word radiation commonly causes anxiety in patients, particularly in the setting of a cosmetic procedure such as laser hair removal. Of course, none of the technology discussed in this text is associated with high-energy ionizing radiation. All laser and light source technology, when used for hair removal, emits light in the visible and near-infrared electromagnetic spectrum.

# BASIC PHYSICS

The basic physics of laser technology is quite simple. In an atom, electrons occupy discrete energy levels or orbits surrounding the nucleus. When an atom absorbs a photon of energy, one or more electrons will move to an unstable, higher energy, outer orbit. This energized atom will rapidly release the photon of energy so the electrons can return to the stable, lower energy configuration. Under normal circumstances, the high-energy state electrons spontaneously decay to their resting orbital energy level while simultaneously releasing photons of energy. This spontaneous release of energy is disorganized and random and is known as incoherent light.[1] This incoherent light is utilized for therapeutic purposes with intense pulsed light sources.

In a laser system, more atoms exist in their unstable, higher energy state than in the usual resting energy configuration. This condition is known as *population inversion* and is a necessary requirement for the lasing process to begin. An excited-state electron can be 'stimulated' by a photon of proper energy to undergo orbital decay. In this situation, two photons of identical wavelength and frequency will exit the atom together, traveling in precisely the same direction in phase with one another. This process constitutes the start of the process of *amplification*.

# COMPOSITION OF LASERS

All lasers are composed of four primary components:

(1)   the lasing medium,
(2)   the resonating or optical cavity which surrounds the laser medium and in which the excitation process occurs,
(3)   the power supply or 'pump' that acts as the exciting mechanism to create population inversion, and
(4)   the delivery system, which may be composed of fiberoptics or articulating mirrors.

There are hair removal lasers encompassing both these types of delivery systems. Lasers are generally named for their active medium and can be divided into three general types: solid, liquid, and gas. All currently available hair removal lasers have in their optical cavity a solid active medium.

Some form of excitation is necessary to generate excited electrons and create population inversion.[2] This can be accomplished by several different methods. None of these is particularly relevant to laser hair removal efficacy and so they will not be discussed here.

It is in the optical resonator that the population inversion of excited electrons results in amplification of light produced by stimulated emission. This is due to the effect of mirrors at each end of the resonating cavity which reflect the waves back and forth many times until a sufficient intensity and complete amplification occur. The energy is then released from one end of the tube through a perforation in a partially reflective mirror. A standard lens of predetermined focal length can focus the beam after it leaves the resonator tube, so as to allow delivery to the target. Most of the currently available laser systems emit collimated energy over a preset distance because of this lens.[2] Light source technology, although emitting similar wavelengths as those seen from lasers, does not emit collimated light.

# CHARACTERISTICS OF LASER IRRADIATION

The stimulated emission of laser irradiation gives laser light three unique characteristics. It is:

1. *Monochromatic*: Although the laser light is actually of a narrow wavelength band in a Gaussian distribution around the characteristic wavelength of the laser, for practical purposes it can be regarded as being of a single and discrete wavelength. The wavelength is determined solely by the laser medium present in the optical cavity. This property is very important therapeutically because selective absorption of the laser light by specific chromophores, such as melanin, hemoglobin, or tattoo ink, is wavelength specific.
2. *Coherent*: The waves of light are temporarily and spatially coherent, i.e. the waves are in phase both in time and space. This is analogous to a group of marchers who are marching in step, in parallel rows and columns, and in the same direction.
3. *Collimated*: The light waves are parallel. This is a direct result of spatial and temporal coherence. This highly ordered pattern of the light allows the beam to be propagated across long distances along optical fibres without beam spreading.

# ENERGY FLUENCE

Knowledge of two concepts is required to understand how a given biologic effect is obtained from any laser system. The first concept is that of energy fluence or the amount of energy delivered to a unit area for a single pulse. This calculation is based on the formula:

$$\text{energy fluence (Joules/cm}^2) = \frac{\text{laser output (watts)} \times \text{laser exposure time (seconds)}}{\text{area of delivered laser beam (cm}^2)}.$$

That second concept is that of the spatial average energy fluence (SAEF). This is the total energy delivered to an entire treatment site. This calculation is based on the formula:

19

$$SAEF = \frac{\text{laser output (watts)} \times \text{pulse number} \times \text{laser exposure time (seconds)}}{\text{area of delivered laser beam (cm}^2\text{)}}.$$

An understanding of these terms should allow the standardization of treatment parameters from one laser facility to another.[3]

# BIOLOGIC EFFECTS OF LASERS

## Introduction

Laser hair removal has recently begun to receive great interest because of its non-invasive mode, the minimal treatment discomfort, and the speed of the procedure. This method of treatment is, as discussed below, based on selective photothermolysis.

In order to select a useful laser hair removal system, one must understand how each laser produces its specific biologic effect on tissue. Emitted laser energy has the following characteristics:[3]

(1) The emitted light conforms to the *Grothus–Draper Law*, which states that light absorption is required for an effect in tissue. If there is no light absorption in or around the hair, no effect on the hair will be observed.

(2) Light can be reflected back to the outside from various interfaces of the skin without a clinical effect. The epidermis is responsible for most of the reflection from skin.

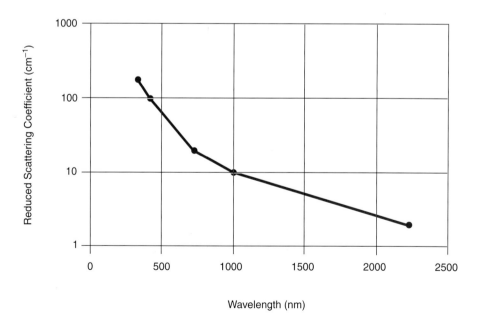

**Figure 2.1.** Effect of wavelength on dermal scattering of light

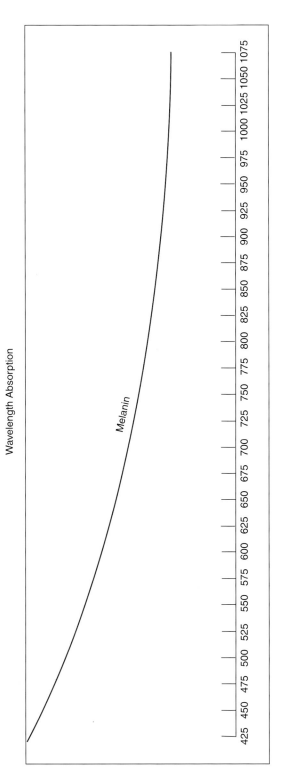

**Figure 2.2.** Melanin absorption curve

21

(3)  Light can be transmitted through the target tissue, such as the dermis, without clinical effect.

(4)  Light can be scattered in all directions away from its primary direction of travel. In skin, dermal collagen is responsible for most light scattering. Forward and sideways scattering will attenuate the fluence of the incident beam with depth. Back scattering may actually increase the fluence within the tissue. The specific contribution of different types of scattering depends on the specific wavelength being used. In general, scattering decreases with longer wavelength. Thus, longer wavelengths penetrate further into the skin (Figure 2.1).

Laser light photons are absorbed by chromophores, which are light absorbing components of the skin. Melanin is the target chromophore in hair although a topically applied carbon chromophore that surrounds the hair has also been utilized. Theoretically other chromophores such as hemoglobin in the vessels surrounding hair could be utilized as well. The chromophore-absorbed energy is converted to thermal energy, with resultant heating of the hair itself.

The specific wavelength of laser light will determine the specific chromophores that will absorb the light energy. Since light is absorbed by hair melanin throughout the visable light and near-infrared spectrum, there are numerous wavelengths that can be effectively utilized for hair removal (Figure 2.2).[4]

## Selective Photothermolysis

The duration of the laser beam's emitted pulse is critical in achieving the desired clinical effect. Heat dissipates from the site of laser absorption mainly by heat diffusion. Large objects lose heat much slower than small objects. There is a defined time period known as the thermal relaxation time, that it takes an object to cool down to the ambient temperature after having been heated. For most chromophores in the skin, this time is determined only by the size of the object. The thermal relaxation time of a melanosome measuring approximately 1µm is approximately 1µs; for hair follicles it is 1–100ms, and for epidermis approximately 3–7ms.

If an object is heated for longer than its thermal relaxation time, there is enough time for thermal diffusion to occur, with resultant heating of surrounding structures. If the pulse duration is far longer than the thermal relaxation time of the target hair and hair follicle, there is heat diffusion and resultant destruction of surrounding structures, with potential risk of scarring.

If an object is heated for a period shorter than its thermal relaxation time, the heat and resultant damage is confined to the target object alone. This dramatically reduces the risk of scarring. Enough energy must be emitted to thermally damage the treated hair without causing excessive damage to areas around the treated hair.

It is this theory of *selective photothermolysis* that states that selective heating is achieved by preferential laser light absorption and heat production in the target chromophore when the pulse duration is shorter than the thermal relaxation time of the target.[5]

# Spot Size

One might think that the spot size of the emitted beam would not be a very important laser parameter. Theoretically, if the spot size is increased and the laser power output is also increased to maintain the same energy fluence, the therapeutic effect would be similar. However, due to sideways laser light scattering in the skin, spot size does make a difference (Figure 2.3). With a small spot size, sideways

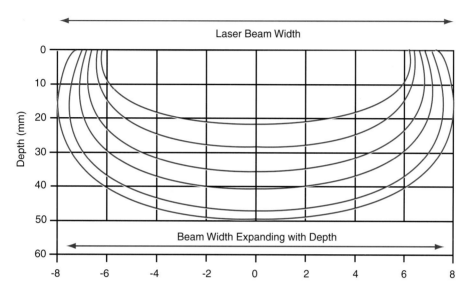

**Figure 2.3.** Effect of laser spot size on depth of laser penetration

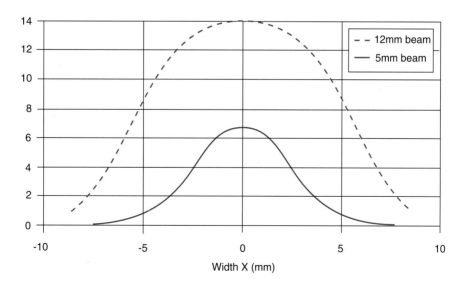

**Figure 2.4.** Relationship between spot size, dermal scattering, and *relative fluence effect*

scattering reduces the energy fluence in tissue far more rapidly than is seen with a large spot size. This effect of spot size is more pronounced at longer and more penetrating wavelengths such as those used with the ruby, alexandrite, diode, and Nd-YAG lasers. A spot size of at least 3–5mm is essential for maximal depth of laser light penetration when treating hair. Using a larger spot size may allow the use of lower fluences. Put differently, the *relative fluence effect* on the skin is greater with larger spot sizes (Figure 2.4). Larger spot sizes, all else being equal, may lead to better hair removal efficacy.

# Wavelength

During the process of laser and light source hair removal, light is absorbed by the absorbing chromophore (usually melanin in the hair shaft and follicle, or topically applied carbon) and converted into heat energy, with a resultant raising of the hair temperature. When the temperature is high enough, irreversible damage may occur to the hair structures. Despite these laser-induced changes, an increase in mutation frequency or DNA damage in cells has not been noted after laser hair removal. Although there is an increase in selective mitochondrial damage, there is no increase in laser-induced free radicals, a marker for cellular mutation damage.[6] Growth of the hair is simply either altered or prevented by laser/light source treatment. Similar hair-altering temperature alterations can be achieved through electrolysis.

When considering the optimal wavelengths for maximal hair removal and minimal epidermal damage, one must consider the process of absorption and scattering of light by different tissues. The primary requirement for choice of emitted wavelengths is that light must penetrate deeply enough into tissue to reach the pluripotential growth center(s) of a treated hair. In the 400–590nm wavelength range, strong absorption by small superficial blood vessels prevents this waveband from penetrating significantly deep enough to have an impact on hair removal. With longer wavelengths there is not only increased dermal penetration but also less dermal scattering. This explains why the ideal wavelengths would appear to be between 600 and 1100nm. Because the epidermis, as well as many of the potentially treated hairs, has high concentrations of melanin, the epidermis is also sensitive to light irradiation. Thus 'selective' photothermolysis and its role in hair removal represent a balance between temperature elevation in the treated hair and in the absorbing epidermis.[7]

There are two types of melanin in hair, depending on hair color. Red and red-blond hair contains greater amounts of phaeomelanin; brown and black hair contains greater amounts of eumelanin. Light absorption of the two types of melanin is different, so absorption depends on the relative concentration of each melanin in the hair.

Although the spectral range of 690–1000nm would appear to be the ideal choice for removing hair that is much darker than the skin, longer wavelengths may be more helpful in damaging deeper hairs that are not much darker than the skin. Conversely, with significant epidermal cooling, one may be able to use slightly shorter wavelengths even when darker skin is treated. Cooling has been accomplished with cold gels, cryogen sprays, and a variety of sapphire-tipped cooling devices.

# Pulse Width

When considering the appropriate timed pulse of delivered energy, one must determine the diameter of treated hairs as well as the depth of penetration of the laser's emitted wavelength. For example, at 694nm, the wavelength of a ruby laser, light penetrates well into and through the dermis. That the laser pulse width is important is explained by the thermal transfer theory.[8] Thermal conduction during the laser pulse heats a region around the site of optical energy absorption. The spatial scale of thermal confinement and resultant thermal, thermomechanical, or thermoacoustic damage is strongly related to the pulse width of the emitted laser irradiation. Q-switched, nanosecond domain laser pulses effectively damage individual pigmented hairs within a hair follicle by confinement of heat solely at the level of the laser-impacted melanosomes. This, at least in an animal model, leads to leukotrichia but not hair loss. Consistent with this concept is the lack of reported permanent human hair loss from the Q-switched ruby, alexandrite, and Nd-YAG lasers despite over a decade of successful clinical experience using these systems to treat tattoos and pigmented lesions. The thermal relaxation time of whole hair follicles is between 1 and 100ms, depending on size. Thermal relaxation times in human terminal hairs have never been measured but have been estimated to be about 10–50ms. Most treated hairs are between 130 and 250µm. In principle, a pulse duration that is shorter than the cooling time of hair, yet longer than the cooling time of the epidermis, should be selected. This will enable the epidermis and small adjacent vessels to cool while the treated hair is being heated. For hair follicles larger than 130µm in diameter, the hair cooling time is longer than the epidermal cooling time (about 3–7ms). Therefore, choosing longer emitted pulses can enhance selectivity. Longer pulse widths, at least in theory, would allow more thermal conduction and damage to non-pigmented regions of the hair follicle but would confine the thermal damage solely to the hair.[8]

# Fluence

The fluences and spot size of treatment also impact on efficacy. Higher delivered energies allow more photons to be delivered to the deeper regions of a hair follicle, thus with laser systems of comparable wavelength, higher fluences usually lead to better results. In addition, when light is applied to the skin, there is scattering of emitted photons. Fluence quickly decays as a function of depth. Thus, most energy is dissipated in radial directions in the more superficial portion of the skin. With larger spot sizes, light penetration becomes more efficient because the delivery of photons becomes more planar. With a more planar distribution, more photons can penetrate more deeply into the treated hair. It is for this reason, as previously described, that a larger spot size, all else being equal, tends to lead to better results.

## Conclusions

As described above, the optimal pulse duration for photothermolysis selective for hair removal would appear to be less than or equal to the thermal relaxation time of the target structure, in this case the treated hair. Simply stated, the thermal relaxation time in seconds of any treated structure is approximately equal to the square of the target diameter in millimeters. Thus for a typically treated hair follicle of 200–300μm in diameter, the thermal relaxation time would be about 40–100ms. In this ideal situation, the laser pulse duration would lie somewhere between the 3–7ms thermal relaxation time of the epidermis and the 40–100ms thermal relaxation time of the treated hair follicle. With such emitted pulses, heat would be extracted from the epidermis during the laser pulse while thermal confinement is kept within the treated hair follicle.

Computer simulations have suggested that:

(1)    the temperature of the irradiated follicle decreases with hair shaft depth,
(2)    using a spot size less than 4 mm could result in light not penetrating deeper than 3mm in depth,
(3)    a black hair shaft follicle of about 50μm in diameter requires a fluence of at least 20J/cm² for coagulation and lighter color hairs require higher delivered energy fluences, and
(4)    thicker hairs require lower energy densities than do thinner hairs.[9]

## REFERENCES

1    Maiman TH. Stimulated optical radiation. Nature 1960;187:4943–9
2    Fuller TA. The physics of surgical lasers. Lasers Surg Med 1980;1:5–14.
3    Anderson R, Parrish J. The optics of human skin. J Invest Dermatol 1981; 88:13–19.
4    Arndt KA, Noe JM. Lasers in dermatology. Arch Dermatol 1982;118:293–5.
5    Wheeland RG, Walker NPJ. Lasers – 25 years later. Int J Dermatol 1986;25:209–216.
6    Haywood R. Ruby laser hair removal. Paper presented at 2nd Annual European Society for Lasers in Aesthetic Surgery, Oxford, England, March 1999.
7    Mainster MA, Sliney DH, Belcher D, et al. Laser photodisruptors. Damage mechanism, instrument design and safety. Ophthalmology 1983;99:973–91.
8    Dierickx CC, Grossman MC, Farinelli WA, et al. Permanent hair removal by normal mode ruby laser. Arch Dermatol 1998;134:837–42.
9    Lask G, Elman M, Slatkine M, et al. Laser-assisted hair removal by selective photothermolysis. Dermatol Surg 1987;23:737–9.

# 3 ELECTROLYSIS FOR PERMANENT HAIR REMOVAL

## KEY POINTS

(1) There are three forms of electrolysis: galvanic, thermolysis, and a blend of the two
(2) Galvanic electrolysis is the more certain method for permanent hair removal but is slower, therefore thermolysis or the blend method are more frequently used
(3) Electrolysis results in the permanent removal of hair

## BACKGROUND

Electrolysis has been used to produce permanent hair loss since 1875 when Dr Charles Michel first used it in St. Louis, Missouri to remove the ingrown hairs of trichiasis.[1] The term *electrolysis* refers to the permanent removal of hair by the insertion of a fine wire needle (probe or filament) into the hair follicle. This needle acts as a conductor to carry the appropriate current to the base of the hair follicle, and particularly to the controlling hair papilla. Some authors[2] have preferred to use the term electroepilation, but the term electrolysis still predominates. The discipline is known as electrology and practitioners are called electrologists. There are three principal methods of performing electrolysis (galvanic electrolysis, thermolysis, and a blend of the two). The goal of each modality is to provide enough electrolysis energy to destroy the germinative matrix cells and the dermal papilla without allowing destructive energy to reach the skin surface. Such a concept, similar to that in laser-induced selective photothermolysis, lessens the risk of unwanted skin surface damage.

# MODALITIES

The three electrolysis modalities and their equipment are standardized and well documented by practitioners, electrologists, equipment manufacturers, regulators, and the medical literature.[3-7]

## Galvanic Electrolysis

In galvanic electrolysis, a direct (galvanic) electric current is passed down a needle into the hair follicle (Figure 3.1). The action of the current causes an interaction between NaCl and $H_2O$ contained within the hair follicle and surrounding tissues. This leads to the formation of lye (NaOH) and hydrogen gas ($H_2$). While the hydrogen gas escapes from the follicle, the NaOH remains (Figure 3.2). Because it is caustic, the NaOH destroys the germinative cells and the dermal papilla. Galvanic electrolysis is the most certain method of electrolysis-induced permanent hair removal. However, it is slow and can require a minute or more of treatment for each hair. Single-needle galvanic electrolysis is not frequently used. However, multiple-needle machines, which can utilize up to 16 needles simultaneously, are popular with a minority of electrologists. Most electrolysis devices advertised for home use are battery operated galvanic (direct) current devices. In experienced hands, they are safe and effective but slow.

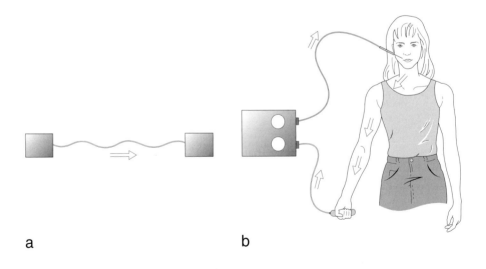

a          b

**Figure 3.1.**   Negatively charged electrons flow from the negative to the positive pole (a) along a wire conductor and (b) in a direct current galvanic electrolysis

28

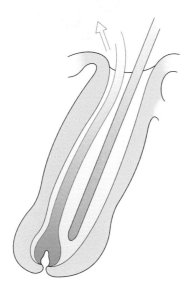

**Figure 3.2.** Lye (NaOH) forms in a straight hair follicle

# Thermolysis

Thermolysis has also been known as short-wave, radio-frequency diathermy and was previously designated under a variety of trade names such as the old *Kree method*, named after the Kree manufacturing company. In this method, passage of a high-frequency current down the needle produces destructive heat in the follicular tissues by molecular vibration (Figures 3.3 and 3.4). This heat then destroys the hair structures and dermal papilla. Thermolysis is much faster than galvanic electrolysis and requires only a few seconds. In high-speed 'flash' thermolysis the higher energy current is applied for only a fraction of a second. The flash method is best used with insulated needles, which protect the upper hair follicle and permit higher energy directly into the lower follicle.

A Japanese variant of thermolysis is the Kobayashi–Yamada insulated needle method, first described in 1985 by Dr Toshio Kobayashi.[8,9] In his method, the thermolysis machine uses energy up to seven times more powerful than that of standard machines. The destructive power is great enough to destroy distorted follicles and hair in all stages of the hair cycle (anagen, catagen, and telogen). The skin surface is protected by 1mm of insulation on the base of the needle. This method is used in several Japanese clinics.

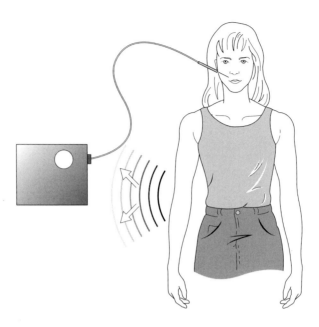

**Figure 3.3.** Capacitative return in a high frequency alternating current in thermolysis

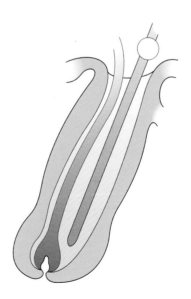

**Figure 3.4.** High frequency alternating thermolysis current stimulates molecules to vibrate, producing destructive heat

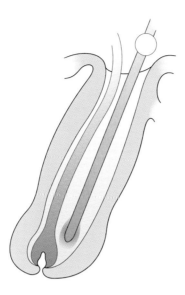

**Figure 3.5.** The blend: heat and lye work together to produce destruction

## The Blend Method

Arthur Hinkel and others developed the blend method in the late 1940s. They were not only the first to describe the blend method but were also the first to explain all aspects of electrolysis is scientific detail.[10] The blend method combines galvanic electrolysis (for sureness) and high frequency thermolysis (for speed). In the blend method heat produced from thermolysis heats up the sodium hydroxide produced by galvanic electrolysis and this increases efficiency. The blend method is a widely used modality (Figure 3.5).

## SHAVING PRIOR TO ELECTROLYSIS

Shaving 1–5 days before electrolysis greatly increases efficacy because it ensures that only growing anagen hairs are treated. This may be particularly important in some areas, such as the arms, legs, thighs, and pubic area, where as many as 80% of hairs may be in telogen (see Table 1.1). Telogen hairs are difficult to permanently eradicate because precise needle insertion is difficult and because the matrix cells and papilla are in a quiescent stage. Because the telogen follicle is so short there is a much greater

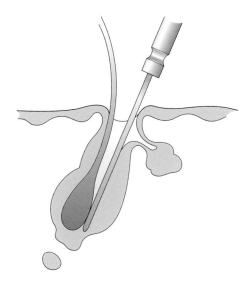

**Figure 3.6.**  Undesirable needle insertion into a telogen hair follicle

risk of destructive energy being delivered closer to the skin surface and therefore undesirable side-effects such as discomfort and superficial skin damage are more likely to occur (Figure 3.6). Although many individuals are resistant to shaving, it should be emphasized to clients that shaving has no effect on hair growth.[11–13]

# PROCEDURE

Usually, prior to electrolysis, the skin is swabbed with a cleanser such as Savlon (chlorhexidine gluconate 1.5% and cetrimide 15%). However, no controlled studies have demonstrated a need for this procedure. Many practitioners prefer to use soap and water. Either way, make-up should be removed prior to electrolysis. People undergoing electrolysis may assume any position; however, for ease and by convention, most clients lie on an electrolysis couch. Three diopter magnifiers are the usual lighting. Standardized electrolysis equipment, including disposable needles, is readily available from electrolysis suppliers.

Precise needle insertion is the cornerstone of electrolysis excellence. Attention must be paid to needle direction, angle, and depth (Figure 3.7). In the specialty of electrolysis, treatment energy is defined as the intensity × duration of the delivered current. Modern computerized machines make it simpler to produce hair destruction by the correct combination of intensity and duration of the current. Regardless of the electrolysis method utilized the goal is to deliver sufficient

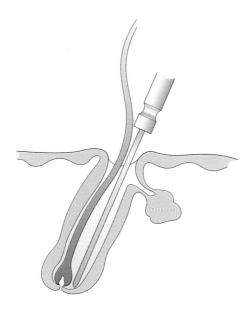

**Figure 3.7.** Correct needle insertion into an anagen hair follicle

current (intensity) for an adequate time (duration) to destroy the growing portion of the hair follicle. As with laser-induced hair removal, there are a variety of combinations and permutations that can lead to good results. However, if the intensity ('fluence', in laser terms) is too high, skin damage may occur. If the intensity is too low, there may not be sufficient energy to destroy the hair root. The same principle applies to duration ('pulse duration', in laser terms). There is no 'always perfect' combination of intensity and duration. One can use any combination of intensity and duration that is appropriate, as long as the combination results in enough treatment energy to destroy the hair roots without producing unwanted side-effects.

When electrolysis is undertaken in an appropriate manner, no resistance should be felt when the hair is removed with gentle forceps traction. The hair bulb should be present. If the hair does not come out easily with gentle forceps traction then it is being plucked rather than destroyed by electrolysis.

As noted above, there are no precise units of measurement available for treatment energy. However, programmable computerized machine manufacturers have built-in relative value scales of treatment energy based on a combination of intensity × duration. For example, one programmable computerized machine has a treatment energy scale of 0–125 units. An average hair would require 50–60 units. One may select a certain number of units that represents the treatment energy and also select an appropriate intensity. The machine automatically calculates the duration required producing that end point. Many machines guide the electrologist by setting the appropriate energy for fine, intermediate, or coarse hairs. The electrologist then observes the clinical response before making fine adjustments to establish a precise working point.[7] After the completion of electrolysis, an electrologist has no way of knowing that the germanitive cells have been destroyed. As mentioned earlier, the best evidence available is that the hair is sufficiently loosened to allow gentle forceps traction removal with an intact hair bulb. Unfortunately, with all methods, there will always be a percentage of regrowth. The post-electrolysis regrowth rate has been estimated to be 20–40%. It is important, however, to distinguish between apparent regrowth and actual regrowth. 'Apparent regrowth' is the appearance of hairs, in the treated area, which in fact never received electrolysis (previous telogen hairs or new hair growth activated by hormonal stimulation). 'Actual regrowth' is the growth of hairs that have been previously treated with electrolysis. The most common causes of actual regrowth are inaccurate insertions, inaccurate intensity, inadequate duration, curved or distorted follicles, and/or insertions into telogen follicles.

## After-Effects, Side-Effects and Patient Comfort

After the completion of electrolysis the skin may or may not be swabbed again with a skin cleanser according to individual preference. Some clients apply nothing whereas others like the feel of witch hazel, a product that has been traditionally used by electrologists for its soothing, cooling effect. Many electrologists apply an aftercare cream such as 0.5% hydrocortisone. Most people are able to return immediately to their regular activities after electrolysis. Some will develop mild post inflammatory erythema and occasional welting. In most, this disappears within a few minutes to an hour. In those few sensitive patients who develop significant erythema or mild folliculitis, the use of 1% hydrocortisone cream with equal parts Polysporin Cream (polymyxin B sulfate and gramicidin) has been found to be helpful. When electrolysis is performed appropriately, small crusts may develop only in a small percentage of cases. These usually heal in a few days. Crusting and other side-effects occur more frequently during the initial sessions until the skin becomes acclimatized and correct intensities and duration are established. Postinflammatory hyperpigmentation may occur in dark-skinned individuals. This usually fades over the ensuing weeks or months. Most people who undergo electrolysis have no significant problems. Complications are generally found only in those with extremely sensitive skin or in those who continue to pluck, wax, manipulate, or otherwise irritate their skin, at the same time as undergoing electrolysis.

Scarring should be extremely unusual after properly performed electrolysis. My colleagues and I have not observed scarring in over 145,000 hours of electrolysis performed in our clinic. Most of the scarring previously attributed to electrolysis actually resulted from inappropriate plucking or picking or other inappropriate interference with the skin. Nevertheless, if electrolysis currents are applied at too high a level, because of operator error or machine defect, scarring can occur.

Electrolysis may be performed on patients of any age but children may not wish to cooperate. There are no limitations with regards to body sites, hair size, or hair colors. Electrolysis is safe in diabetics, in those on gold or other drug therapy, and in those immunocompromised by disease or drugs. Electrolysis should not be performed in areas of inflamed or diseased skin. Most modern pacemakers are not affected by the passage of the electrolysis electric current; however, patients with pacemakers should check with their cardiologist and/or the pacemaker manufacturer before proceeding with electrolysis.

Electrolysis needles are very fine (Figure 3.8). In the first 40,000 hours of electrolysis in my clinic, we have documented only two broken needles in the skin. These did not produce any long-term sequelae. We suspect that this problem probably occurs more frequently than is recognized. For all methods, rigid pointed needles should be avoided because flexible needles with a bulbous tip are easier to thread into curved follicles and are less likely to pierce the base of the follicle (Figure 3.8). Accurate needle insertion, the establishment of an appropriate working point, and the appropriate combination of intensity and duration to deliver the treatment energy are more important than the specific modality utilized (i.e. galvanic electrolysis, thermolysis, or blend). (Figures 3.7 and 3.9).

There is a degree of warmth or burning discomfort with electrolysis; most patients find it tolerable. Some body areas such as the upper lip are particularly sensitive. The pre-application of ice-packs is helpful in reducing discomfort but the introduction of EMLA (eutectic mixture of local anesthetics) has lessened many sensitivity problems.[14]

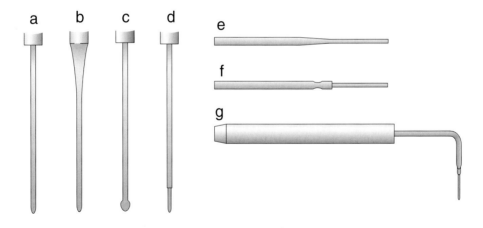

**Figure 3.8.** Various needle types: (a) straight; (b) tapered; (c) bulbous; (d) insulated; (e) one piece; (f) two piece (blade crimped inside shank); (g) Kobayashi–Yamada. 1, 1.00mm insulation; 2, 3.00mm non-insulated piercing tip

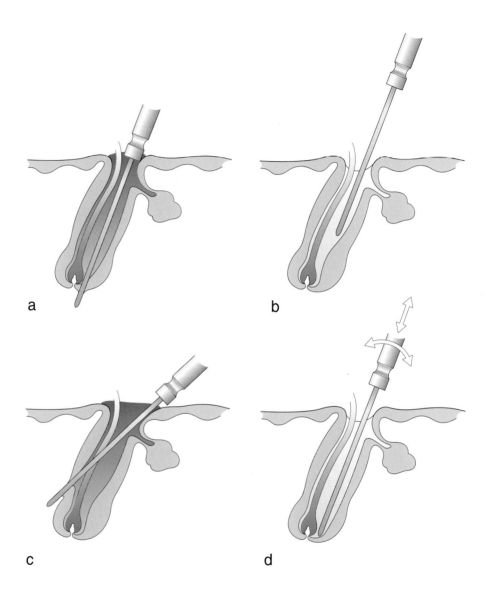

**Figure 3.9.** Examples of poor insertions: (a) insertion too deep; (b) too shallow; (c) incorrect angle of insertion (may lead to rupture through follicular wall); (d) needle motion when insertion is completed

# Length and Number of Sessions

When using the blend method or regular thermolysis the number of hairs removed per hour varies between 150 and 300 depending on the type of hair, the subject's tolerance, and operator speed. Hair removal is much slower if there are ingrown hairs or other problems. The number of hairs removed in the flash thermolysis method is greater. However, unless this technique is limited to very fine hairs there will be more regrowth. Galvanic electrolysis is much slower than the other methods requiring from 15 to 180 seconds for treatment of each hair. Galvanic electrolysis is often reserved for very coarse hairs.

The length of an electrolysis treatment session will also vary with the size of the hairs, the hair density of the area being treated, the tolerance of the client. For example, a few hairs on the chin or upper lip will only take 5–15 minutes to remove while extensive hair on the face or extremities can take 3 or more hours. Most individuals acclimatize to the electrolysis procedure. The length of their sessions usually increases with experience. Electrolysis sessions may be held as frequently as is practical for both the electrologist and the client. However, if the skin shows redness or other problems it should not be retreated until the inflammation has resolved.

The average peri- or postmenopausal woman with a few hairs on the chin requires three to six visits of 15–30 minutes duration. Ordinarily several visits are required during the first month or two of treatment. Later, several more visits can be used to treat regrown or previously untreated telogen hairs. Ordinarily one or two visits per year would be required thereafter. An individual with dense hair in the mustache area might require a 15–30 minute session weekly for about 6 months, and approximately every other week for the next 6 months. This would be followed by treatments once a month during the next year. Occasional maintenance sessions would be required during the next few years. Hair in the axillary regions tends to be more stable. Clearing the axillae in an average person usually takes 3–8 hours with permanent removal requiring 20–40 hours. Permanent hair removal of a few unwanted hairs around the nipples will take a total of 1–5 hours of electrolysis at appropriate intervals. Dense hairs on the arms, legs, and back will take many hours of electrolysis for their total removal. Treatment of these areas is often impractical except in the most committed individuals.

Electrolysis is ideal for localized areas of hair removal. The areas most commonly treated in women are the face, eyebrows, breasts, the lower abdomen, inner thighs (bikini area), and the axillae. Men most frequently wish to have hair removed from between the eyebrows, around the ears, in areas where ingrown hairs are a problem (the beard area), and the upper back and shoulders.

# INITIAL CLEARING VERSUS PERMANENT REMOVAL

Initial clearing is defined as the removal of visible hair. For example – electrolysis can clear an average (preshaved) leg of hair in about 8 hours. However, about 80% of leg hairs are in the telogen stage. Such hairs may not be visible. Therefore, a single electrolysis session (much like a single laser session) only impacts on about one-fifth of the hairs. Even with expertly performed electrolysis there is a regrowth rate of 20–40%. In addition, in individuals with hormonal abnormalities, new hair follicle growth may be activated in androgen-sensitive areas; this will necessitate a further increase in the number of treatment sessions required.

# RESULTS

The histologic findings after electrolysis are well documented. Several biopsy studies have shown its effectiveness in destroying the dermal papilla and the depths of the hair follicle.[5,7] A properly treated hair will not regrow. Most investigators believe that the dermal papilla must be destroyed if electrolysis is to lead to permanent hair removal. This issue (see Chapter 1) has been further complicated by the recent work suggesting that, in the mouse, hair follicle stem cells reside in the bulge area of the hair follicle.[15] Most investigators believe that there is an essential epidermal–mesodermal interaction. Controversy exists as to whether or not the papilla, or bulge area, is paramount.[16–18]

Urushibata et al.[19] studied 14 healthy adult Japanese women and demonstrated that there was total regrowth after plucking axillary hairs but no hair regrowth after electrolysis. Richards and Meharg[6] observed the effects of 140,000 hours of electrolysis in women with hirsutism and found that electrolysis helped control the hirsutism; 93% of the women were improved. However, in hirsutism, dormant hair follicles are continually being activated. They noted that for the best results electrolysis must be combined with treatment of excess androgen production. The same principles presumably apply to laser hair removal.

# LACK OF DISEASE TRANSMISSION BY ELECTROLYSIS

Millions of electrolysis hours have been performed since the introduction of this procedure in 1875. There has never been a report of disease transmission. In the literature, there have only been three accounts of health complications associated with electrolysis; these have been widely cited. I do not believe them to be of concern but they are discussed below.

Petrozzi[20] described a patient whose plane warts were spread by electrolysis. Scratching, shaving, or other trauma such as electrolysis can spread infectious lesions, such as plane warts or herpes. Electrolysis should not be performed in abnormal skin. Cookson and Harris[21] reported the case of a woman who developed endocarditis while receiving electrolysis. This in all likelihood was a coincidental occurrence. The association had never been reported previously and has not been since. There is no scientific evidence that there is enough manipulation in electrolysis to induce bacteremia. There are no reports that establish any causal relationship whatsoever between electrolysis and endocarditis. A recent report by Ditmars and Maguna[22] described a case of sporotrichosis occurring in a woman who was receiving electrolysis. No details were given; the relationship presumably was coincidental.

# REGULATIONS

Regulations concerning electrolysis, where they exist, vary greatly. Slightly over 50% of the states in the United States require specific electrolysis licensing. Only a physician may practice electrolysis in France or Japan. In many countries there are no regulations.

Electrolysis training requirements also vary. For example, in the United States, they range from 300 hours in Delaware to 1100 hours in Massachusetts.[7]

# ROLE OF ELECTROLYSIS

Despite varying techniques and approaches, electrolysis, as a hair removal technique, has a long record of both safety and efficacy. What role electrolysis plays in the setting of improved laser hair removal techniques remains unclear. Although large areas of hair may be more efficiently removed with lasers, non-pigmented hair appears to respond best to electrolysis. In addition, it may be more economical to treat small areas of undesirable hair with electrolysis than with lasers. In an ideal setting, the two techniques would complement each other.

# REFERENCES

1   Michel CE. Trichiasis and districhiasis with an improved method for their radical treatment. St Louis Clin Rec 1875;2:145–8
2   Richards RN, McKenzie MA, Meharg GE. Electroepilation (electrolysis) in hirsutism: 35,000 hours experience on the face and neck. J Am Acad Dermatol 1986;15:693–7.
3   Wagner RF Jr, Tomich JM, Grande DJ. Electrolysis and thermolysis for permanent hair removal. J Am Acad Dermatol 1985;12:441–9.
4   Hobbs ER, Ratz, JL, James B. Electrosurgical epilation. Dermatol Clin 1987;5:437–44.
5   Kligman AM, Peters L. Histologic changes of human hair follicles after electrolysis: a comparison of two methods. Cutis 1984;34:169–76.
6   Richards RN, Meharg GE. Electrolysis: observations from 13 years and 140,000 hours of experience. J Am Acad Dermatol 1995;33:662–6.

7 Richards RN, Meharg GE. Cosmetic and medical electrolysis and temporary hair removal, 2nd edition. Toronto: Medric Ltd; 1997.

8 Kobayashi T. Electrosurgery using insulated needles: epilation. J Dermatol Surg Oncol 1985;11:993–1000.

9 Kobayashi T, Yamada S. Electrosurgery using insulated needles: basic studies. J Dermatol Surg Oncol 1987;13:1081–4.

10 Hinkel A, Lind RW. Electrolysis, thermolysis and the blend: the principles and practice of permanent hair removal. California: Arroway Publishers; 1968.

11 Trotter M. Hair growth and shaving. Anatom Rec 1928;37:373–9.

12 Saitoh N, Uzuka M, Sakamoto M. Human hair cycle. J Invest Dermatol 1970;54:65–81.

13 Lynfield YL, MacWilliams P. Shaving and hair growth. J Invest Dermatol 1970;55:170–2.

14 Wagner RF, Flores CA, Argo LF. A double blind placebo controlled study of a 5% lidocaine/prilocaine cream (EMLA) for topical anesthesia during thermolysis. J Dermatol Surg Oncol 1994;20:140–50.

15 Cotsarelis G, Sun TT, Lavker RM. Label-retaining cells reside in the bulge area of the pilosebaceous unit: implications for follicular stem cells, hair cycle and skin carcinogenesis. Cell 1990; 61:1321–7.

16 Stenn KS, Combates NJ, Eilertsen KJ, et al. Hair follicle growth controls. Dermatol Clin 1996;14:543–58.

17 Cotsarelis G. The hair follicle. Dying for attention. Am J Pathol 1997;151:1505–9.

18 Olsen EA. Methods of hair removal. J Am Acad Dermatol 1999;40:143–55.

19 Urushibata O, Kase K. A comparitive study of axillary hair removal in women: plucking vs. the blend method. J Dermatol 1995;22:738–42.

20 Petrozzi JW. Verrucae planae spread by electrolysis. Cutis 1980;26:85.

21 Cookson WO, Harris ARC. Diptheroid endocarditis after electrolysis. BMJ 1981;282:1513–14.

22 Ditmars DM, Maguna P. Neck skin sporotrichosis after electrolysis. Plast Reconstr Surg 1998; 101:504–6.

# 4 NORMAL MODE RUBY LASER

## KEY POINTS

(1) Normal mode ruby lasers emit 694nm visible light wavelength
(2) The melanin absorption is the best among all the visible light hair removal lasers
(3) The risk of post-treatment pigmentary changes is greater than with other lasers (unless significant cooling is applied or longer pulse durations are utilized)
(4) Millisecond high fluence systems have been cleared by the US FDA for permanent hair reduction

## BACKGROUND

Leon Goldman MD, the father of laser medicine, was among the first to use a ruby laser (50µs pulse duration) to evaluate the laser-induced damage threshold of pigmented lesions (Figure 4.1). His studies suggested a ruby laser-induced selective effect, perhaps at the level of the melanosome.[1] It was 20 years later that Polla and Dover in separate studies demonstrated that the Q-switched ruby laser targeted individual melanosomes.[2] Electron microscopic analysis of these thermally damaged targeted melanosomes revealed membrane disruption and disorganization of their internal contents. The destruction of melanosomes appeared to be pulse-width dependent. Pulse durations of both 40 and 750ns disrupted melanosomes. This is consistent with the theory of selective photothermolysis, which states that the pulse duration of an emitted laser wavelength must be less than the thermal relaxation time of the targeted object. A typical 1.0µm melanosome has a thermal relaxation time somewhere around 1.0µs.[3]

The specific cause of melanosomal destruction is unknown. Plasma probably does not form. The peak powers produced by lasers interacting with melanosomes are

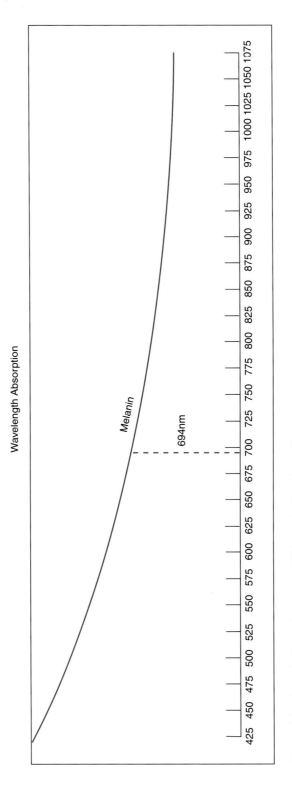

**Figure 4.1.** Melanin absorption curve of 694nm ruby laser irradiation

quite low for such an occurrence. Shockwave and/or cavitation damage, the photomechanical physical effects produced from thermal expansion, and/or the extreme temperature gradients created within the melanosome are the more likely explanations. Studies of acoustic waves generated by pulsed irradiation of melanosomes and pigmented cells support these possibilities. Melanin absorbs and localizes the high-intensity irradiation from Q-switched lasers, thereby creating a sharp temperature gradient between the melanosome and its surrounding other structures. This gradient leads to thermal expansion and the generation and propagation of acoustic waves, which can mechanically damage the melanosome-laden cells.

Tissue repair following laser-induced melanosomal disruption demonstrates a two-stage initial transient cutaneous depigmentation followed by subsequent regimentation weeks later. Black guinea-pig skin, irradiated with 40ns Q-switched ruby pulses at radiant exposures of 0.4J/cm$^2$ or greater, whitens immediately, fades in 20 minutes, depigments 7–10 days later, and then repigments 4–8 weeks after treatment. Of note is the fact that the repigmented guinea-pig skin displays a persistent leukotrichia that can last up to 4 months after laser irradiation.[3] Despite the promising results seen in guinea-pig hair, such results have not been seen in human hair after treatment with a nanosecond Q-switched ruby laser. It has been assumed that a nanosecond Q-switched laser pulse, although causing photomechanical destruction of a hair, does not cause enough photothermal damage to lead to long-term changes in hair. Instead, it has been postulated that a longer millisecond laser pulse is required.

# CLINICAL STUDIES

Normal mode millisecond ruby lasers produce 694nm red light. This 694nm laser light is well absorbed by melanin-containing hair. Adrian has evaluated the hair removal efficacy of a 1ms ruby laser. In this study, 50 subjects were treated twice and evaluated 3 months after the second treatment. Adrian noted 100% hair regrowth at the end of the study. In addition, extensive epidermal blistering was seen after treatment (R Adrian, personal communication). This early study showed that while 694nm laser irradiation is well absorbed by both epidermal and follicular melanin, the 1ms pulse duration was too short to lead to significant thermal damage of follicular melanin.

More recently, a number of studies on the use of ruby lasers to remove hair have been published. In the rest of this section, the studies are discussed in detail.

# Grossman et al.[4]

In the first published study evaluating the use of a ruby laser on human hair, Grossman, et al. used a 270μs pulsed 694nm system at 1Hz. The laser contained a contact cooling device that was designed to maximize delivery of light to the deeper portions of the hair follicle while minimizing epidermal damage. This contact device contained a sapphire lens that was cooled to 4°C. Such a device provides heat conduction from the epidermis before, during, and after each laser pulse. The laser energy was delivered through a 6mm spot size.

Thirteen human volunteers (12 men, 1 woman) were treated. All had Fitzpatrick skin phenotypes I–III; all had brown or black hair. Treated areas were the back or thigh. Eight $3 \times 2$cm sites were chosen on each subject. Before laser treatment, half the sites were shaved while the remaining sites were epilated with a commercially available cold wax. One shaven site and one wax-epilated site served as untreated control sites. The treated sites were evaluated using fluences of 30, 40, and 60J/cm². Hair counts were determined 1, 3, and 6 months after laser treatment. Hair regrowth was defined as the percentage of terminal hairs present after treatment, as compared with the number before treatment.

Immediately after treatment, all sites became erythematous and edematous. There was rare purpura, epidermal whitening, and/or epidermal ablation. In evaluating the 1, 3, and 6 month results, the authors noted a statistically significant growth delay at 1 and 3 months for all utilized fluences at both shaven and epilated sites in comparison with the unexposed shaven and epilated control sites. At 6 months there was significantly less hair only at the 60J/cm² shaved sites.

Hyperpigmentation, present in three subjects, had cleared by the 6-month follow-up visit. Two subjects had transient hypopigmentation; no scarring was noted.

Biopsy specimens revealed laser-induced damage to the follicular epithelium. Hair shafts were fragmented. There was little histologic difference between the sites treated with 40J/cm² and those treated with 60J/cm². The biopsy results showed thermal coagulation and asymmetric focal rupture of the follicular epithelium. The focal rupture suggested that laser-induced steam formation occurred, with temperatures exceeding 100°C in portions of the hair follicle.

The authors noted that the presence of a hair shaft was not absolutely necessary for temporary hair removal. This effect resulted from the ample melanin contained in both the follicular epithelium and papilla. At 6 months, however, there was significant hair loss only at *shaven* sites treated with the highest fluences. This suggests that the presence of a hair shaft actually enhances selective photothermolysis.

Based on their data, the authors concluded that temporary hair removal was not fluence dependent. Permanent hair loss, however, may require a greater damage threshold.

Of the 13 subjects in the study, 7 were followed up to 2 years after laser exposure.[5] At 1 year and 2 years after laser treatment, 4 of the 7 still had obvious hair loss confined to the laser treated sites and 3 had complete or nearly complete hair regrowth. In all 7 participants, there was no significant change in terminal hair counts 6 months, 1 year, and 2 years after laser exposure. It should be noted that the best results were noted at the highest fluences (60J/cm²). The major significance of this study was that it showed that 'permanent' terminal coarse hair removal was possible after a single treatment with a high-fluence normal mode ruby laser. The fact that hair counts were unchanged 6 months after laser treatment suggests that 6-month follow-up may be sufficient to determine final results of laser hair removal.

This study further evaluated what appear to be two distinct laser hair removal responses – that of temporary growth delay and that of permanent hair loss. Temporary growth delay would appear to be caused by laser damage inducing the telogen phase. Permanent hair loss would appear to be associated with miniaturization of hair follicles. These findings were seen in all 13 treated subjects. Furthermore, in all subjects, whether or not permanent hair loss was noted, there was a growth delay consistent with the length of telogen. The presence of a hair shaft during laser treatment was not required to induce growth delay. Such findings, as discussed in the original study, were seen at all fluences in both shaved and wax-epilated sites. However, permanent hair loss, after a single laser treatment, was only noted where there *was* a hair shaft. Thus, permanence would be expected in pretreatment shaved individuals, but not in pretreatment epilated patients.

It should be noted that the authors treated hair only on the thigh and trunks of their subjects. On the thigh up to 70% of hairs are in telogen at any given time. Thus, those hairs that appeared to be resistant to laser treatment may have been in the telogen phase at the time of exposure. Multiple treatments would, therefore, be expected to lead to better results.

The authors, in evaluating histologic findings, looked at both terminal and miniaturized vellus-like hairs. Of note was that the total number of hairs in laser-treated areas remained the same as in the control non-treated areas. However, in the laser-treated sites, there was a reduction in the number of large terminal hairs, with a corresponding reciprocal increase in the number of small vellus-like hairs. Such a hair is defined as one that has a cross-sectional hair shaft diameter of less than 30μm. This is consistent with anecdotal clinical findings of thinner, lighter hairs after laser treatment. Because the size of a hair depends on the size of the papilla and hair bulb, ruby laser pulses would appear to miniaturize both the papilla and bulb, either by direct photothermal injury or by injury to other follicle structures that control formation of the bulb during each anagen cycle.

# Lask et al.[6]

Lask et al. evaluated a ruby laser with pulse duration of 1.2ms in the treatment of dark hair on the arms of 20 subjects. All areas were treated once at 25–40J/cm², with a 4–5mm spot size. Pretreatment cooling was accomplished by the use of a 0°C transparent cooling gel. Minimal post-treatment erythema was reported; it resolved within 3–4 days. In this study 20–60% of the hair was absent after the 3-month evaluation. These findings, suggestive of a temporary growth delay, were consistent with the findings of Grossman et al.[4] The authors suggested that improved results would be expected after more than one treatment session. With this approach, an increasing number of previously untreated anagen hairs would be treated.

## Williams et al.[7]

Williams et al. published hair removal data after three treatments using a 3ms ruby laser with a sapphire-tipped cooling device. Forty-eight sites in 25 adults (13 men, 12 women) with Fitzpatrick skin phenotypes I–III were evaluated. All had blond, brown, or black hair. Treated sites included the face, back, shoulder, lower leg, bikini, and axillae. Subjects were treated with either a 7 or 10mm handpiece, with fluences varying between 10 and 40J/cm². As a general rule, lower fluences were utilized for darker complexions to lessen epidermal blistering.

This was the first published study evaluating the efficacy of multiple ruby laser treatments. The authors expected that multiple treatments would lead to improved results. Hair regrowth was measured at 4 weeks after the first treatment, 4 weeks after the second treatment, and 16 weeks after the third treatment.

In the immediate post-laser period, most subjects showed the expected mild edema and perifollicular erythema. No purpura was noted. Although 2 patients with Fitzpatrick skin phenotypes I–III showed hyperpigmentation at 10 days post-treatment, this hyperpigmentation was resolved at 3 months. Almost all subjects with the aforementioned skin phenotypes were noted to have the expected treatment-induced hypopigmentation lasting 1–10 days after laser treatment. No subjects were reported to have scarring or any pigmentary changes 4 months after the third treatment.

The authors also evaluated the relationship between skin type, treatment fluence, and percentage of hair regrowth. In the 12 Fitzpatrick skin phenotype I sites treated, the average fluence was 26J/cm². Fitzpatrick skin phenotypes II–III were treated with correspondingly lower fluences (Table 4.1).

It should be noted that although the darker skin phenotypes could only tolerate lower fluences than could those with lighter skin phenotypes, this did not necessarily

| Skin type | No. of sites treated | Average fluence (J/cm²) | % Regrowth after: | | |
|---|---|---|---|---|---|
| | | | 1st Treatment | 2nd Treatment | 3rd Treatment |
| I | 12 | 26 | 63 | 47 | 43 |
| II | 28 | 23 | 68 | 45 | 37 |
| III | 8 | 14 | 62 | 26 | 22 |
| Adapted from Williams et al.[7] | | | | | |

**Table 4.1.** Relationship of skin type, treatment fluence, and hair regrowth

translate into lesser improvement. Also, all treated individuals, of all skin phenotypes, were noted to have an increase in the number of vellus hairs after subsequent treatments. Stated differently, all individuals were noted to have a corresponding increase in vellus hairs with a decrease in the number of terminal hairs. Thus, a state of 'absolute hairlessness' should not be expected.

The authors noted that some anatomic areas responded better to treatment than did others. For example, a lower percentage of hair *regrowth* was observed on the face (1–37%), underarms (23–34%) and trunk (39–57%). This pattern was true irrespective of skin type or hair colour. Such variations could be explained by differences in hair depth at different sites and/or different hair growth cycles in different anatomic areas.

Hair color, as would be expected, had an impact on efficacy of laser treatments. In general, subjects with dark brown or black hair had a lower percentage of hair regrowth after three treatments than did those with light brown or blond hair. This finding is consistent with the theory that melanin is the absorbing chromophore.

# Solomon[8]

Solomon evaluated the treatment responses of 72 patients whose 76 anatomic sites were treated with a 3ms ruby laser. Patients were laser-treated between one to four times. Treatments were given on a monthly basis. Although the author indicated that three different fluences were utilized, the exact parameters were not well defined in this study. The author utilized forceful compression of the skin during treatment, to flatten the dermis and reduce the amount of blood in the skin. This was intended to decrease the distance between the laser-emitted pulse and the depths of the hair. Whether this approach truly leads to better results has not been proved. Anatomic areas of treatment included the face (42 patients), back (10), arms (4), axillae (2), shoulder (2), breasts (1), abdomen (1), legs (3), and bikini area (11). The patients were followed between 3 and 6 months after the last treatment (average follow-up was 3.5 months).

Seventy-one of 72 patients responded to treatment. However, the authors were unable to assess the duration of hair loss. Although no patients were noted to be completely hair free, all reported less presence of hair than they had experienced after the conventional modalities they had used before. Hypopigmentation lasting up to 6 months was noted in 2 patients. Hyperpigmentation occurred in 4 patients. Scarring was not noted in any treated individuals. All patients who had had previous electrolysis found ruby laser treatment less painful. Unfortunately, this study is difficult to evaluate because of the lack of well-defined treatment parameters. However, it can be said with certainty that temporary hair loss was induced by the ruby laser treatment.

# Bjerring et al.[9]

Bjerring et al. evaluated the results of ruby laser hair removal in 133 patients; 98% of the patients were women. The median age was 43 years (range 8–78 years). All patients had light complexions, although some were tanned. Hair colors included blond, red, brown, black, and gray. Ruby laser pulse durations were 700–800µs. Utilized fluences were 10–25J/cm². Treated areas included the upper lip, cheek, chin/neck, abdomen, thigh, and bikini area. The average number of treatments was 2.2 (range 1–9). No cooling was applied to the skin prior to treatment. The authors judged success in two ways: (1) greater than 50% hair removal after 90 days, and (2) greater than 25% removal after 90 days.

With success defined as greater than 50% hair removal, 59% of the patients reported successful results for 90 or more days. With success defined as greater than 25% removal after 90 days, 75% of patients reported successful treatment. When evaluating patient satisfaction, the results were somewhat disappointing. Only 33.5% of patients were very satisfied. This is consistent with the finding that hairiness is determined not only by hair counts, but also by length, width, density, and darkness of hairs. Of note in this study was the observation that the anatomic site had no influence on the percentage of successful hair removal. This was in contrast to the findings of Williams et al.[7] In addition, anatomic site had no effect on the overall result of subjective evaluation of treatment.

The more gray hair was present in the pretreatment sites, the lesser was the response noted. The authors observed that when the percentage of gray hair was less than 50% (thus, dark hairs represented more than 50% of the hairs), 69% of treated patients experienced successful hair removal after 90 days. The success rate decreased to 42% among patients with more than 50% gray hair. When successful, hair removal was defined as more than 25% hair removed after 90 days: patients with less than 50% gray hair experienced successful treatment in 79% of cases, whereas patients with more than 50% of gray hair showed success 70% of the time.

The authors found that only 'slight' discomfort was experienced by 72% of the patients, while 28% found the procedure to be moderately or very painful. In comparing ruby laser hair removal with other forms of epilation, 80% of individuals said laser treatment was either less painful or no more painful than electrolysis.

Only 35% of treated individuals were noted to have erythema and a flare reaction immediately after treatment. Most clinicians feel that some sort of perifollicular erythema and edema is required for optimal results. Thus, the authors' results might have been improved had a greater inflammatory reaction been seen in all treated individuals. In 98% of the subjects, all swelling and erythema had disappeared within 48 hours. In 64% there was a brownish discoloration of the skin immediately after treatment. This was presumably due to the vaporization of hair after treatment, and is commonly seen after laser treatment with all visible light lasers. The median duration of the discoloration was 5 days. In addition, 14% of the patients were noted to have 'true' postinflammatory hyperpigmentation and 10% showed evidence of hypopigmentation. At 90 days, none of the patients showed evidence of postinflammatory hyperpigmentation, while 1 patient had persistent hypopigmentation. Finally, the authors noted that previously electroepilated or tweezer-treated, scarred areas needed higher delivered laser energies for successful therapy. This was presumably due to the lower light transmission and greater horizontal scattering through scarred tissue.

By their own admission, it is difficult to interpret these authors' data. The distribution of hairs as well as the duration of hairs in anagen/telogen phases will vary from site to site. The authors suggested that observations should best be evaluated by anatomic site or alternatively at the end of an entire anagen/catagen/telogen cycle.

# McCoy et al.[10]

McCoy et al. have recently further evaluated the scientific basis of ruby laser-induced hair response. They treated 24 subjects with a 3ms ruby laser. All hairs were brown or black, and all hair was from the axilla or groin. Subjects avoided all significant forms of epilation for 1 month prior to the trial. There were two phases to the trial.

In Phase 1 of the study, 15 of the 24 subjects were treated *once*, with five different fluences: 10, 15, 20, 30, and 40J/cm². Biopsies were taken immediately after treatment, 1 week later, or 4 weeks later. In Phase 2 of the trial, the remaining 9 subjects were treated on *three* successive occasions with three different fluences: 20, 30, and 40J/cm². Representative biopsies were taken after one, two, and three treatments.

In Phase I, immediate post-treatment biopsies showed damage to the hair shaft. The severity of damage appeared to be fluence related. Although cell viability appeared to be lost in the inner root sheaths, outer root sheaths remained viable at all fluences except 40J/cm². The epidermis and dermis were unaffected at all utilized fluences.

One-week biopsies showed changes consistent with those of early catagen. At 1 week, cellular death was noted in the outer root sheaths, with pigment incontinence and degeneration of melanocytes. The severity of changes was fluence related. Telogen and vellus hairs appeared to have been unaffected by laser irradiation. Although the epidermis remained normal, the dermis showed a low-grade inflammatory infiltrate.

At 4-week biopsy, follicular changes consistent with late catagen and early telogen stages of hair growth were noted at all treated fluences. At this point, the dermis had returned to normal.

Phase 2 biopsies, performed 8 weeks after one treatment, revealed both terminal and vellus hairs at all utilized fluences. Although the terminal hairs were noted to be in either the anagen or late catagen/telogen stages, more hairs were in the second phase than would normally be expected. These findings were similar at all utilized energies.

At 6 weeks after two treatments, separated by 12 weeks, findings consistent with cystic dilatation and terminal hair plugging of the infundibulum were noted. The deeper dermis revealed follicles in both telogen and anagen. No hair shafts were noted to protrude from the follicular orifices.

After three treatments, 6-week biopsies showed all terminal hairs to be in late catagen/early telogen or in early anagen phases.

The authors postulated that the progressive histologic changes seen after repeated treatments are consistent with the improved clinical results seen after several treatments.

## Dierickx et al.[11]

Dierickx et al. evaluated the required fluences of a 3ms ruby laser for both temporary and permanent hair removal. They noted that 80% of patients could show permanent hair reduction, but the response was fluence dependent. Temporary hair removal could be seen in all individuals and with all hair colors. However, even temporary hair removal required a fluence of at least 5J/cm$^2$. Histologic findings immediately after treatment were consistent with apoptosis. One day later, further apoptosis and catagen induction was noted. One week later minimal cellular death was noted. Finally, at 1 month, the normal apoptotic cellular death consistent with the natural involution of the lower two-thirds of the catagen follicle was noted.[11]

## Silva-Siwady[12]

Silva-Siwady evaluated hair removal efficacy of a 1.2ms ruby laser in Hispanic patients. 187 subjects (average age of 30 years) were evaluated. All subjects were treated at least three times. Subjects with Fitzpatrick I–II phenotypes were treated at 30–35J/cm$^2$. Subjects with Fitzpatrick phenotypes III–IV, as would be expected, were treated with lesser fluences of 20–25J/cm$^2$. Treatment intervals were 4–8 weeks on the face and neck and 6–12 weeks on the arms, backs, and legs. All subjects were evaluated 4–17 months after the final treatment.

Silva-Siwady noted that at least 50% of skin phenotype I–II individuals showed more than 70% hair loss at the end of the study. Fewer than 30% of the phenotype III–IV individuals were noted to have lost more than 70% hair loss at the end of the study. This disparity may be due to the lower fluences utilized in the subjects with darker complexions. Alternatively, epidermal melanin may be competing with follicular melanin in these individuals.[12] These findings were different from those seen by Williams et al.[7]

## Elman[13]

Elman also evaluated ruby laser side-effects in darker-skinned Israeli patients.[13] She compared 1.2 and 20ms ruby lasers. Both pulse durations were delivered through a cooling gel. Immediately after treatment, slight erythema was noted at the 1.2ms sites while none was seen at the 20ms sites. At 15 minutes after treatment, loss of pigmentation was noted at the 1.2ms sites; there were no pigmentary changes at the 20ms sites. At 1 day, a crust was noted at the 1.2ms sites; slight loss of pigmentation was noted at the 20ms sites. The findings were the same at 8 days. At 17 days, hypopigmentation was noted at the 1.2ms sites, while only minimal hyperpigmentation was noted at the 20ms sites. Her conclusion was that, with all factors being equal, longer pulse durations might be safer in patients who have darker complexions.

# Anderson et al.[14]

Anderson et al., in a 10-site multicenter study, evaluated hair removal efficacy in 183 patients (30 men, 153 women) given up to six treatments during the course of 1 year. All body sites were represented, and skin types I–V were included. A 694nm, 3ms ruby laser was delivered with a 7 or 10mm spot size and a sapphire cooling device. Subjects were treated with the highest fluence tolerated, with a range of 10–60J/cm². All were evaluated at baseline and 6 months after the final treatment. All body sites except eyelashes were treated. Retreatments were undertaken at 6 to 12 week intervals depending on degree of hair regrowth.

Of the 183 initially treated subjects, 142 were ultimately evaluated. Eighty per cent were treated with a 7mm spot size with fluences between 20 and 60J/cm². Twenty per cent were treated with a 10mm spot size with fluences between 10 and 24J/cm². The mean number of treatments was 4.5. There was 100% hair loss in the treatment area in 19% of the subjects, regardless of the number of treatments, body sites, skin type, or hair color. Only 2% had less than 25% hair loss or total regrowth. The mean treatment fluence for subjects with 100% hair loss at the 6-month follow-up was 32J/cm² (range 20–40J/cm²). After a single treatment, 67% of subjects showed greater than 50% hair loss in the treated area. After multiple treatments, the percentage of subjects with greater than 50% hair loss increased to 90%. The majority of subjects had greater than 75% hair loss at 6 months after the final treatment. After a single treatment, most subjects showed no change either in color or texture of hairs. However, by the final 6-month follow-up visit, more than 90% of subjects showed finer hair and greater than 80% had lighter hair. The greatest response was noted in the axilla and bikini region, while the thighs and upper lip showed the poorest response.

No scarring or textural changes were noted, although 6% of treated individuals were reported to have hyperpigmentation at 6 months. The incidence of hypopigmentation was 3%. Histologic evaluation noted showed miniaturization of treated hair follicles.

# Lieu[15]

Lieu, in evaluating histologic changes, after 900μs ruby laser irradiation, noted intracellular vacuoles in basal epidermal cells with an intact dermal–epidermal junction. Significant damage to melanin was noted. However, not all hair follicles were damaged. Normal appearing hairs were interspersed with damaged hairs. In addition, most hair bulbs were not damaged. Although the follicular bulb depth in this study averaged 2.47mm, the depth of laser-induced damage, although somewhat fluence related, varied in a narrow range between 1.34 and 1.49mm. This depth of laser-induced damage was consistent with the assumption that it is the bulge, not the bulb, that is more significantly damaged after laser treatment.

## Lin et al.[16]

Consistent with Lieu's study, Lin et al. have suggested a treatment strategy for ruby laser hair removal. They noted that anagen phase hair follicles were particularly sensitive to damage from ruby laser pulses. The authors assumed that this occurred because anagen phase melanin pigmentation is needed to provide the chromophore for selective photothermolysis. They suggested that a second treatment be given at about the same time as the hair begins to appear on the skin surface. It would be at this time that early anagen hairs would be more superficial in the dermis and therefore more susceptible to laser-induced damage. Although such a theory is plausible, it has yet to be proved.

# AVAILABLE RUBY LASER SYSTEMS

## EpiLaser (Coherent/Palomar Medical)

The EpiLaser is a normal mode (non-Q-switched), pulsed 694nm ruby laser. The currently available system delivers a 3ms pulse with fluences ranging between 10 and 75J/cm$^2$ through either a 7 or 10mm handpiece. A specially designed contact cooling handpiece consisting of an actively cooled glass sapphire prism system is used to deliver a convergent beam with a 20mm focal length to the skin. This cooling handpiece is firmly held against the surface before, during, and after each pulse of light to minimize thermal injury to the pigmented epidermis. Cooling at 0°C also maximizes laser intensity in the deeper dermis. Finally, the cooling lessens patient discomfort.

Treatment is performed by delivering light in a continuous pattern at 0.5Hz with 3ms adjacent pulses delivered with the cooling handpiece held firmly in contact with the skin. Overlapping of pulses does not appear to be harmful. The range of energy fluences used for effective treatment may be from 20J/cm$^2$ for darkly pigmented individuals up to 50J/cm$^2$ or higher for fair-skinned individuals.

## EpiTouch (ESC/Sharplan, Norwood, MA)

The EpiTouch is a normal mode ruby laser that can also be used in a Q-switched nanosecond mode for the treatment of tattoos and pigmented lesions. This laser removes hair in a manner much like that seen with the EpiLaser. This system uses a cooling transparent gel to minimize reflectance and scattering of the delivered beam. The cooling also lessens thermal injury to the epidermis. A template is used to allow precise treatment of all hairs in a particular area. The parameters for this system are 1.2ms pulses at 0.8Hz with a 4- to 6mm beam diameter. Delivered fluences vary from 20 to 40J/cm$^2$ (Figure 4.2).

## E-2000 (Palomar Medical Technologies, Lexington, MA)

This is the second-generation ruby laser system from this company. It is improved from the EpiLaser in several ways. The laser light is delivered through a fiber-optic system rather than an articulated arm, making it more user friendly. A pulse duration of 3ms, much like that in the EpiLaser, can be utilized. In addition a 100ms pulse

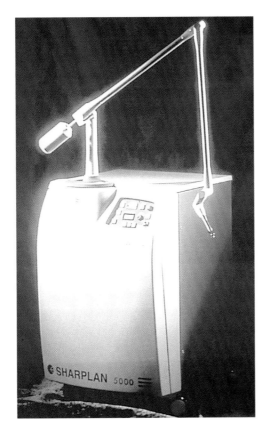

**Figure 4.2.** EpiTouch ruby laser

duration can be used. Use of the longer pulse duration is suggested for greater safety in darker-skinned individuals. Such a pulse duration many also be more effective for the treatment of thicker hairs. Fluences up to 50J/cm$^2$ are available. The sapphire-tipped cooling device is cooled to –10°C which also leads to greater epidermal cooling in individuals with darker complexions. Spot sizes of 10 × 10mm and 20 × 20mm are available; the laser fires at 1Hz (Figure 4.3).

## Medilas R (Dornier MedTech, Germany)

This ruby laser is unique for its flexible fiber in a 1–3 Hz system. Fluences of up to 30J/cm$^2$ can be obtained with 7–10mm spot sizes. Pulse durations of up to 5ms are available (Figure 4.4).

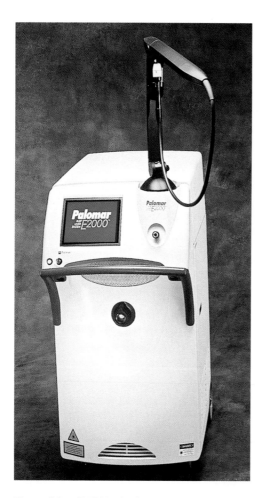

**Figure 4.3.**   E-2000 ruby laser

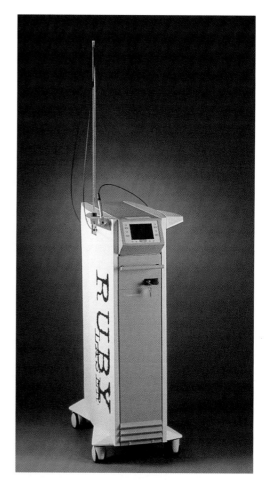

**Figure 4.4.**   Medilas R ruby laser

## EpiStar (Aesculap)

This ruby laser, much like the EpiTouch system, can be used in both a Q-switched and a normal pulsing mode. The normal mode delivered pulse duration is 2ms; fluences delivered through a 7mm spot size are 25–40J/cm². Unlike the other ruby lasers, this system is marketed with a scanning device.

# MY APPROACH

I have found all of the ruby lasers to be very useful in removing unwanted hair and treating hair-induced folliculitis in Fitzpatrick I and II skin phenotypes. Unless appropriate cooling is utilized, Fitzpatrick skin phenotype III and even sun-tanned type II individuals tend to have postinflammatory pigmentary changes (Figures 4.5 to 4.41). This may be lessened, when a ruby laser such as the E-2000 is used, with a –10°C cooling device (Figures 4.42 to 4.44). Alternatively, cooling can be provided by use of cooling gels. When gels are used, they must be replaced often enough so as to prevent their being warmed by contact with human skin. There are no currently marketed ruby lasers that utilize a cryogen spray as a cooling modality.

The treatment technique commences with preoperative shaving of the treatment site. This reduces treatment-induced odor, prevents long pigmented hairs that lie on the skin surface from conducting thermal energy to the adjacent epidermis, and promotes transmission of laser energy down the hair follicle. A small amount of post-treatment crusting and erythema is to be expected. In darkly pigmented or heavily tanned individuals, it may be beneficial to use topical hydroquinones and meticulous sunscreen protection for several weeks prior to treatment in order to reduce inadvertent injury to epidermal pigment. Individuals with recent suntans should not be treated until pretreatment hydroquinones have been used for at least 1 month. Postinflammatory pigmentary changes still are to be expected in individuals who have darker complexions.

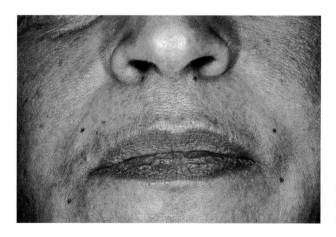

**Figure 4.5.** Upper lip hair before treatment with a ruby laser

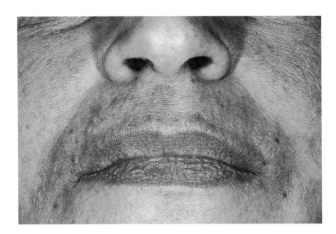

**Figure 4.6.** Upper lip immediately after treatment with a ruby laser. Note mild crusting

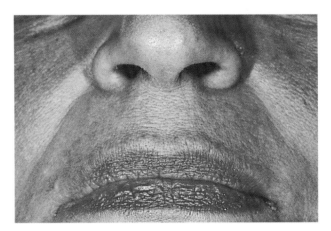

**Figure 4.7.** Upper lip 3 months after one session of ruby laser treatment

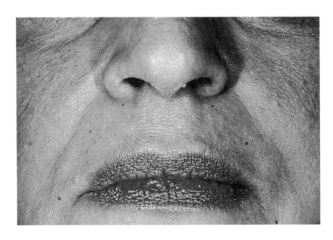

**Figure 4.8.** Upper lip 4 months after two sessions of ruby laser treatment

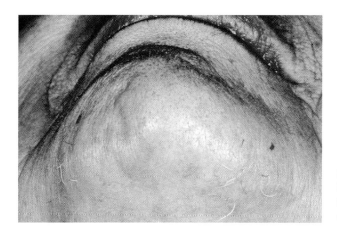

**Figure 4.9.** Chin hairs before ruby laser treatment. Note presence of dark and white hairs

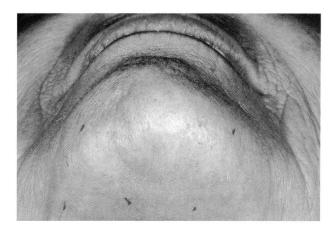

**Figure 4.10.** Chin 1 month after ruby laser treatment. Note transient absence of white hairs

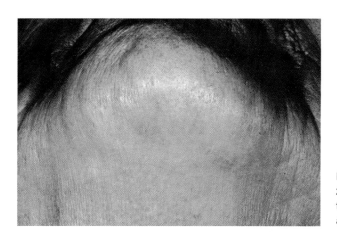

**Figure 4.11.** Chin 2 months after ruby laser treatment. Note transient absence of white hairs

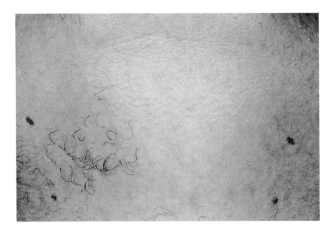

**Figure 4.12** Curly thickened chin hairs before ruby laser treatment.

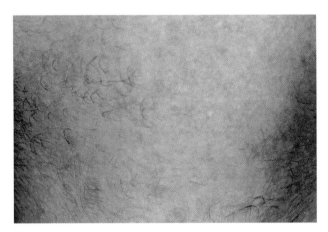

**Figure 4.13** Curly thickened chin hairs 3 months after one ruby laser treatment. Note almost all hairs have regrown.

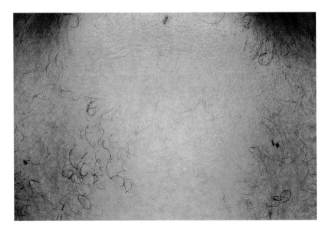

**Figure 4.14** Chin hairs 4 months after three ruby laser treatments. Note hairs are thinner and less dense.

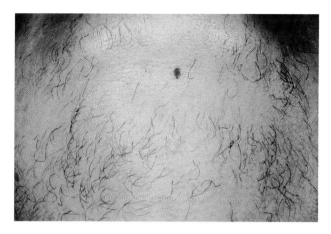

**Figure 4.15.** Hirsute woman with thick, dense chin hairs

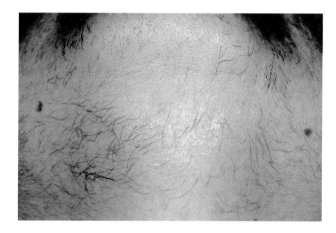

**Figure 4.16.** No change 3 months after one treatment with ruby laser

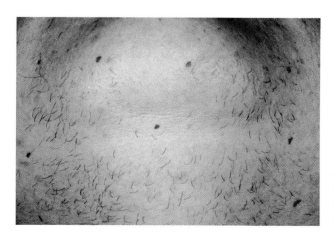

**Figure 4.17.** Slight thinning of hair and lessened hair density 3 months after two ruby laser sessions

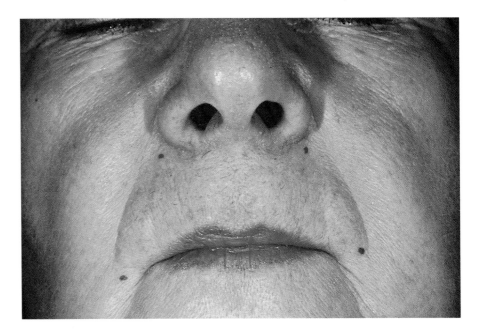

**Figure 4.18.** Upper lip hairs in a postmenopausal woman before ruby laser treatment

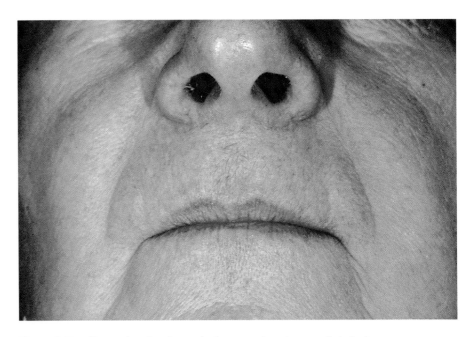

**Figure 4.19.** Six months after three ruby laser sessions to upper lip hairs in a postmenopausal woman. Note near absence of hair

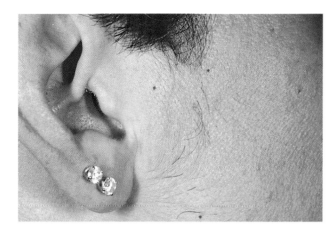

**Figure 4.20.** Right cheek hair before ruby laser treatment

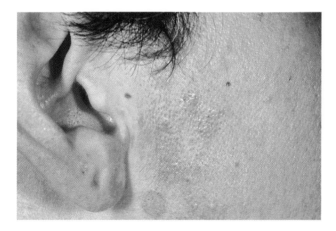

**Figure 4.21.** Mild crusting of right cheek skin immediately after ruby laser treatment. This is to be expected

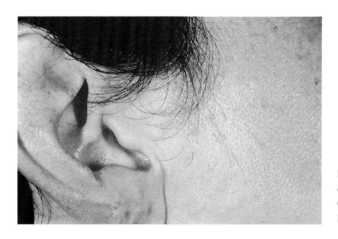

**Figure 4.22.** Thinning of right cheek hairs 6 months after four ruby laser sessions

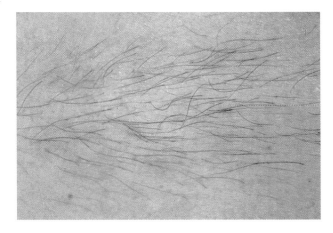

**Figure 4.23.** Chest hairs in a hirsute woman before ruby laser treatment

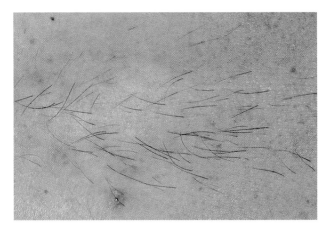

**Figure 4.24.** Chest hairs in a hirsute woman 3 months after three ruby laser sessions

**Figure 4.25.** Near absence of chest hairs in a hirsute woman 6 months after six ruby laser sessions

**Figure 4.26.** Persistent small area of hypopigmentation 4 months after a Fitzpatrick skin phenotype IV individual was treated with a ruby laser

**Figure 4.27.** Female abdominal hairs prior to treatment with a ruby laser

**Figure 4.28.** Near absence of abdominal hairs 8 months after three ruby laser sessions

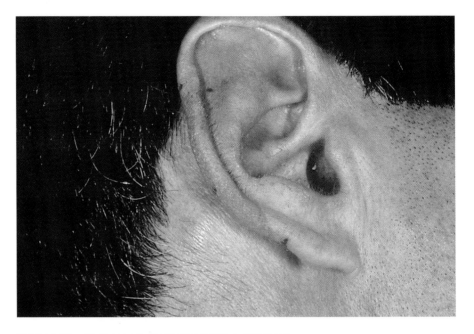

**Figure 4.29.** Male ear prior to treatment with a ruby laser

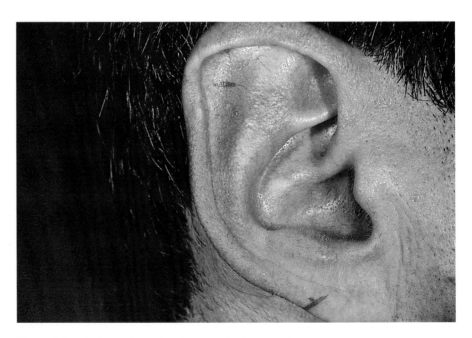

**Figure 4.30.** Male ear 3 months after one ruby laser session

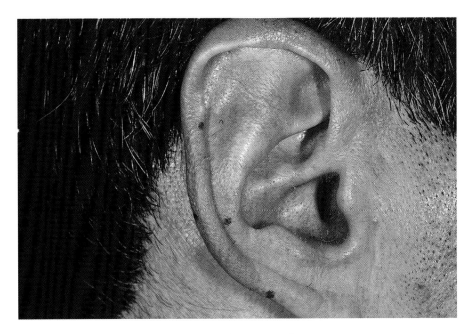

**Figure 4.31.** Male ear 3 months after two ruby laser sessions

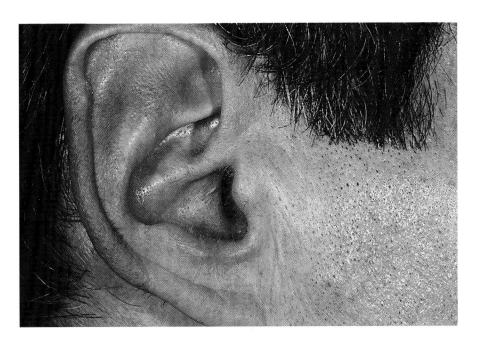

**Figure 4.32.** Male ear 6 months after three ruby laser sessions. Note persistence of fine hairs

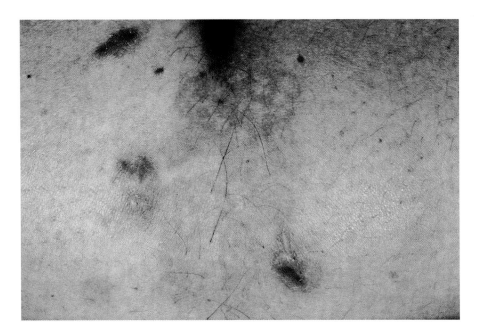

**Figure 4.33.**   Folliculitis and hair prior to treatment with ruby laser

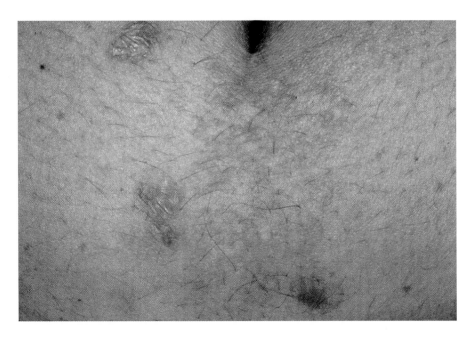

**Figure 4.34.**   Thinning of hair and improved folliculitis after ruby laser treatment

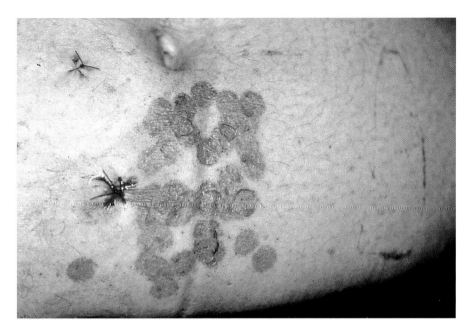

**Figure 4.35.** Significant blistering immediately after ruby laser treatment at 40J/cm$^2$. A lesser fluence must be utilized for treatment

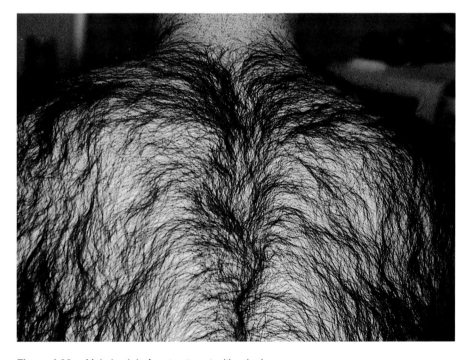

**Figure 4.36.** Male back before treatment with ruby laser

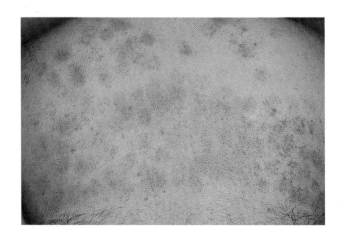

**Figure 4.37.** Postinflammatory hyperpigmentation 2 months after ruby laser treatment

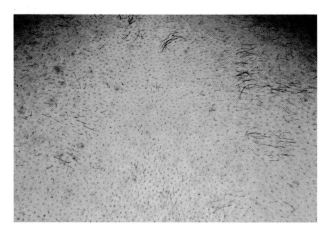

**Figure 4.38.** Three months after first ruby laser session

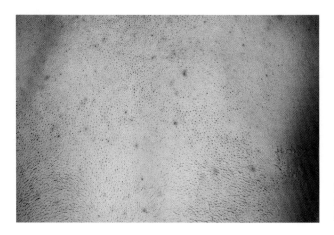

**Figure 4.39.** Three months after second ruby laser session

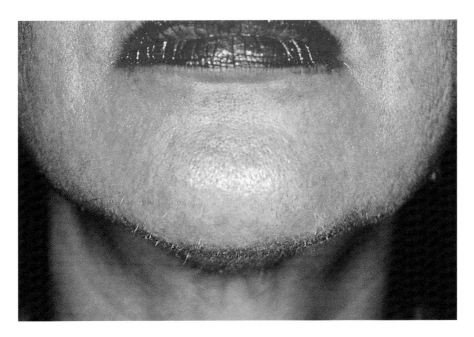

**Figure 4.40.** Postmenopausal woman with black and white chin hairs

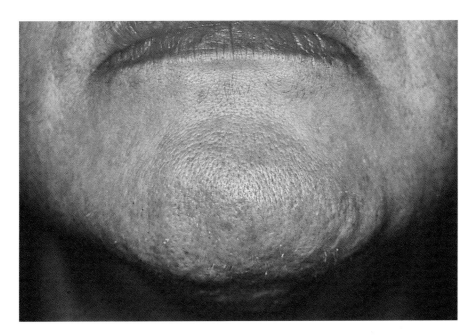

**Figure 4.41.** Five months after three ruby hair removal sessions. Note excellent response in dark hairs and minimal response in white hairs

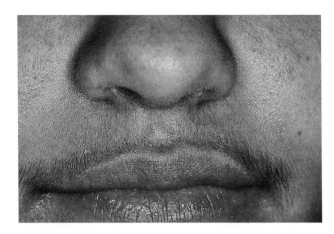

**Figure 4.42.** Fitzpatrick skin phenotype IV before ruby laser treatment

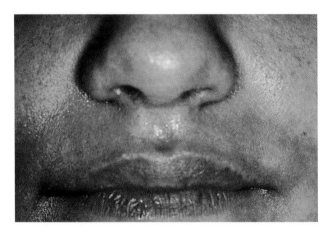

**Figure 4.43.** Immediately after ruby laser treatment using 100ms pulse and −10°C cooling to protect epidermis

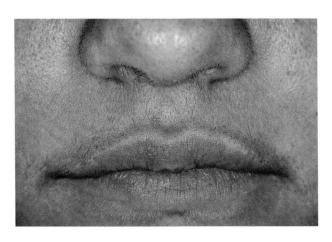

**Figure 4.44.** Four months after second treatment with ruby laser using 100ms pulse and −10°C cooling to protect epidermis

Ruby lasers, when used with almost all fluences, can lead to temporary hair loss at all treated areas. However, choosing appropriate anatomic locations and using higher fluences will increase the likelihood of permanent hair reduction after multiple treatments. Even though permanent hair loss is not to be expected in all individuals, lessening of hair density and thickness is a common finding.

The ideal treatment parameters must be individualized for each patient, based on clinical experience and professional judgment. For individuals who have darker complexions, the novice might consider delivering the laser energy in several individual test pulses at an inconspicuous site with an energy fluence of $20J/cm^2$. The delivered energies are then slowly increased. Undesirable epidermal changes such as whitening and blistering are to be avoided.

Prolonged and permanent hair loss may occur following the use of all normal mode ruby lasers; however, great variation in treatment results is often seen. Most patients with brown or black hair obtain a 2- to 6-month growing delay after a single treatment. There is usually only mild discomfort at the time of treatment. Pain may be diminished by the use of topical or injected anesthetics.

Transient erythema and edema are also occasionally seen and irregular pigmentation of 1–3 months duration is often noted. No permanent skin change, depigmentation, or scarring has thus far been reported in the literature. However, there are now anecdotal cases of rare laser-induced scarring and such a risk must be recognized.

There is more accumulated data about the ruby laser's hair removal efficacy than there is for any other hair removal system. However, as will be seen in subsequent chapters of this book, the information derived from ruby laser studies appears to be quite similar to the early evidence derived from research on hair removal by alexandrite and diode lasers and intense pulsed light (i.e. non-coherent light).

# REFERENCES

1   Goldman L, Blaney DJ, Kindel DJ, et al. Effect of the laser beam on the skin: preliminary report. J Invest Dermatol 1963;40:121–2.
2   Polla LL, Margolis RJ, Dover JS, et al. Melanosomes are a primary target of Q-switched ruby laser irradiation in guinea pig skin. J Invest Dermatol 1987;89:281–6.
3   Goldberg DJ. Q-switched ruby laser treatment of benign pigmented legions of the skin. J Dermatol Surg Oncol 1993;19:251–3.
4   Grossman MC, Dierickz C, Farinelli W, et al. Damaged to hair follicles by normal-mode ruby laser pulses. J Am Acad Dermatol 1996;35:889–94.
5   Dierickx CC, Grossman MC, Farinelli WA, Anderson RR. Permanent hair removal by normal-mode ruby laser. Arch Dermatol 1998;134:839–42.
6   Lask G, Elman M, Slatkine M, et al. Laser-assisted hair removal by selective photothermolysis. Dermatol Surg 1997;23:737-9.
7   Williams R, Havoonjian BS, Isagholian K, et al. A clinical study of hair removal using the long-pulsed ruby laser. Dermatol Surg 1998;24:837–42.

8    Solomon MP. Hair removal using the long-pulsed ruby laser. Ann Plas Surg 1998;41:1–6.

9    Bjerring P, Zachariae H, Lybecker H, Clement M. Evaluation of the free-running ruby laser for hair removal. Acta Derm Venerol (Stockh) 1998;78:48–51.

10   McCoy S, Evans A, James C. Histological studies of hair follicles treated with a 3-msec pulsed ruby laser. Lasers Surg Med 1999;24:142–50.

11   Dierickx C, Campos VB, Lin WF, Anderson RR. Influence of hair growth cycle on efficacy of laser hair removal. Lasers Surg Med 1999;24(suppl 11):21.

12   Silva-Siwady JG. Ruby laser hair removal. Presented at Eighth International Symposium on Cosmetic Laser Surgery. New Orleans, USA, March 1999.

13   Elman M. Hair removal with a very long pulse (20msec) ruby laser. Presented at Eighth International Symposium on Cosmetic Laser Surgery. New Orleans, USA, March 1999.

14   Anderson R, Burns AJ, Garden J, et al. Multicenter study of long-pulse ruby laser hair removal. Lasers Surg Med 1999;24 (suppl 11):21.

15   Lieu SH. Ruby laser hair removal. Second Annual European Society for Lasers in Aesthetic Surgery, Oxford, England, March 1999.

16   Lin TD, Manuskiatti W, Dierickx CC, et al. Hair growth cycle affects hair follicle destruction by ruby laser pulses. J Invest Dermatol 1998; 111:107–13.

# 5 NORMAL MODE ALEXANDRITE LASER

## KEY POINTS

(1) Normal mode alexandrite lasers emit 755nm visible light/near-infrared wavelength

(2) There is excellent melanin absorption, albeit somewhat less than ruby lasers

(3) The risk of post-treatment pigmentary changes is slightly less than with ruby lasers (risk is lessened if significant cooling is applied or when longer pulse durations are utilized)

(4) High fluence systems should lead to similar permanent hair reduction as seen with some ruby lasers.

(5) The fiber-optic delivery systems are user friendly

## BACKGROUND

The Q-switched alexandrite laser, used for the treatment of pigmented lesions and tattoos, is a solid state laser that emits light at 755nm with pulse durations between 50 and 100ns. Less data has been published on this laser as compared to the Q-switched ruby laser. However, because the wavelength and pulse durations are similar to those of the Q-switched ruby laser, the results are similar. A good response has been seen in the treatment of lentigines and *café au lait* macules. Dermal pigmented lesions, such as nevus of Ota, also respond. The 755nm wavelength of this laser penetrates deeply enough to effect the growth centers of hair. In fact, the longer the wavelength, the deeper the penetration. Thus, alexandrite laser wavelengths although not as well absorbed by melanin as those of the ruby wavelengths, do penetrate more deeply into the dermis (Figures 5.1 and 5.2). Nevertheless, as with the Q-switched ruby lasers, there are no documented cases of long-term hair removal induced by Q-switched alexandrite lasers.

When Q-switched alexandrite lasers are used to treat either pigmented lesions or tattoos, short-term hair removal can be seen. However, the nanosecond pulses of

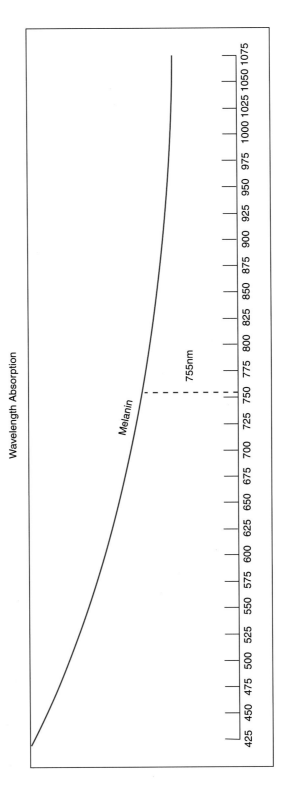

**Figure 5.1.** Melanin absorption curve of 755nm alexandrite laser irradiation

74

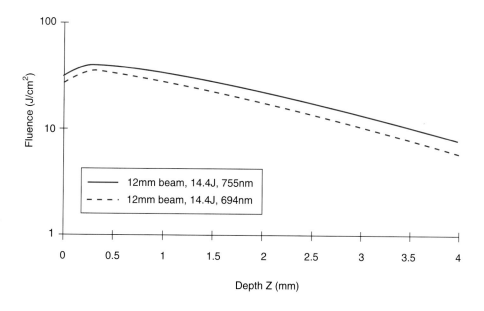

**Figure 5.2.** Relationship between fluence and dermal penetration depth of alexandrite 755nm (solid line) and ruby 694nm (dotted line) irradiation

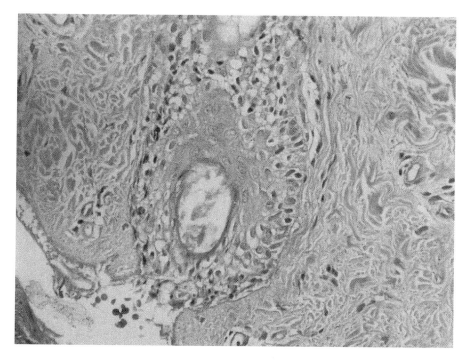

**Figure 5.3.** Distinct vacuolization of hair follicle immediately after treatment with an alexandrite laser

these systems are not long enough to induce the photothermal damage necessary for effective permanent changes in hair. Normal mode non-Q-switched millisecond pulse duration alexandrite lasers do cause the requisite selective hair follicle damage for acceptable results (Figure 5.3).

When the alexandrite laser's longer wavelength is compared with 694nm ruby laser irradiation, we find that less light is scattered as it passes through the dermis, compared with ruby laser irradiation (Figure 5.2). There may also be less risk of epidermal damage, due to the slightly lower epidermal melanin absorption, compared with the ruby wavelength.

# CLINICAL STUDIES

As already stated, the number of published studies on use of alexandrite lasers is limited. Studies carried out to date are reviewed in this section.

## Finkel et al.[1]

Finkel et al. were among the first groups to evaluate the efficacy of the alexandrite laser in removing unwanted hair. They treated 126 patients (10 men, 116 women) with a 2ms alexandrite laser. Among the 116 female patients, 77 individuals had facial hair treated (full face – 25; sideburns – 12; upper lip – 15; chin – 25); 15 individuals had bikini and leg hair treated; 4 individuals had axillae hair treated; 10 individuals had areolar hair treated; 10 individuals had abdominal hair treated. The 10 male patients had backs and/or chests treated. The study was undertaken over a 15-month period.

All subjects were treated with a 2ms alexandrite laser at 20–40J/cm$^2$ (average of 25J/cm$^2$) with a 7mm spot size and 5 pulses per second. Cooling of the epidermis was accomplished with a topical cooling gel. The total number of treatments varied between three sessions on the sideburns, bikini line, legs, and areolar areas of the breast, and five sessions on the upper lip. Treatment intervals varied between 1 month on the upper lip and 2.5 months on the sideburn and chin. The interval between treatments was 1.5–2.0 months for the bikini region, axillae, men's backs and chests, areolar breast hair, and abdomen. The authors noted light erythema in 10% of treated patients. The erythema lasted up to several days. Superficial burns, and blistering, were noted in 6% of individuals. Hypopigmentation lasted up to 3 months.

The average hair count taken before a second treatment was 65% of the hair at baseline. However, the numbers of hair varied in different anatomic areas. Fifty per cent of the hair was removed from the axillae, periareolar, and sideburn regions; 30% of the hair was removed from the full face, bikini area, leg, men's back and chest, and abdomen regions; 20% of the hair was removed from the upper lip and chin regions.

As would be expected, there was progressive improvement with each hair removal session. The average amount of hair present 3 months after the final treatment was markedly less than seen after the first session. An average of only 12% of hair persisted at the final analysis. The results varied from 95% of hairs removed from the sideburns; 90% of hairs removed from the upper lip, bikini, legs, axillae, and periareolar breast area; 85% of the hairs removed from the chin, male backs and chest areas; and 75% of the hairs removed from the abdomen.

The authors found that treatment with this particular 2ms alexandrite laser was extremely fast because of the 5 pulse per second repetition rate. They also noticed that it was important to avoid creating the expectation of permanent hair removal.

It should be emphasized that the complications reported in this study, although minimal, might be lessened by using a strict regimen of epidermal cooling prior to treatment. This can at times be difficult with topical cooling gels.

# Woo et al.[2]

These authors treated some 392 patients with a 20ms alexandrite laser and noted 44–58% hair loss 1 month after one treatment session. It is difficult to draw any conclusions from such a short follow-up period except that short-term hair removal is possible with the system utilized in this study.

# Narukar et al.[3]

Of greater interest was a study by Narukar et al. which evaluated both a 20 and 5ms pulse duration alexandrite laser in skin phenotypes IV–V. All individuals were treated with less than $20J/cm^2$. In this study, better results were obtained with the 20ms pulse duration. Thus, longer pulse duration systems may be more beneficial in darker skinned individuals.[3]

# Nanni and Alster[4]

The findings of Narukar et al. must be contrasted with the observations of Nanni and Alster. They also evaluated the hair removal efficacy of different alexandrite laser pulse durations. They noted that the ideal laser parameters and treatment candidates for photoepilation remain largely unknown. In their study, they examined the hair removal clinical efficacy and side-effect profile of a 5, 10, or 20ms duration pulsed alexandrite laser[4].

Thirty-six subjects (9 men, 27 women, age range 18–68 years, average age 31 years) were evaluated. Only terminal hairs were treated. Hair was treated from the upper lip, back, or lower extremities. All subjects had Fitzpatrick skin phototypes

I–V. A total of 36 anatomic locations (4 upper lips, 7 backs, and 25 legs) were treated. Hair colors included brown and black in 32 subjects, gray in 4 subjects, and blonde in 2 subjects.

All areas to be treated were cooled with a thin film of cooled gel. Fluences of 15–20J/cm² (average of 18J/cm²) were delivered. Comparisons were made between the 5, 10, and 20ms pulse durations. Exposed hair shafts were completely vaporized upon laser impact, with evidence only of residual shaft remnants in the follicle. An immediate erythematous skin response was an observed end-point in the laser-irradiated sites.

All laser-treated areas displayed a significant delay in hair regrowth compared with a control area at 1 week and 1 and 3 months. No significant differences in hair regrowth rates were seen between the use of 5, 10, and 20ms pulse durations. An average of 66% hair reduction was recorded at the 1-month follow-up, 27% average hair reduction was observed at the 3-month follow-up, and only a 4% hair decrease remained at the 6-month follow-up visit. The authors noted that after the one treatment utilized in this study, there was on average no significant reduction in hair growth by the 6 month follow-up. Nevertheless, three individual subjects did experience a cosmetically visible reduction in hair density (hair reductions of 11, 20, and 18%) during this time period. These subjects were all noted to be Fitzpatrick skin phenotype III with brown hair. All had received treatment to their lower extremities.

Complications were limited to immediate post-treatment erythema in 97% of treated sites, minimal intraoperative treatment pain in 85%, transient hyperpigmentation in 3%, and mild blistering in less than 1% (1 case) of treated subjects. Of note was the fact that although hyperpigmentation was observed at all pulse durations in certain individuals, it was generally of less severity and resolved more rapidly in the areas treated with a 20ms pulse duration. These findings were consistent with those seen by Narukar. The average duration of hyperpigmentation was 6 weeks.

The authors noted that all pulse durations resulted in equivalent hair removal. However, they acknowledged that this result might be due to the small sample size studied. Another plausible explanation is that laser hair removal efficacy is similar using a variety of millisecond pulse durations.

It is theoretically possible that a 20ms pulse duration alexandrite laser could be less traumatic to epidermal melanosomes than is a shorter pulse duration system. Small cutaneous targets, such as melanosomes, being more severely damaged by shorter laser pulses, would explain this. Larger cutaneous structures such as hair follicles, however, sustain greater injury at longer pulse durations. This is due to the longer time required for laser energy to be absorbed by these structures. An enhanced selectivity by the longer 20ms pulse duration, therefore, might be best observed in study subjects who exhibited very mild post-treatment erythema and hyperpigmentation. What was not determined in this study was whether a slightly shorter pulse duration might be more effective in thinner hair and a correspondingly longer pulse duration might be more effective in thicker larger hairs.

It should be noted that higher fluences (up to 40J/cm²) are often necessary when the ruby laser is used to achieve long-term hair reduction. Because the alexandrite laser penetrates deeper into the dermis than does the ruby laser, such high fluences may not be required. Nevertheless, the fluences used in this study were conservative and may have led to a reduced rate of efficacy. Higher fluences may be required to maximize potential efficacy.

In Nanni and Alster's study, blonde and gray hairs did not respond as well to alexandrite laser treatment as brown or black hairs. This is due to the reduced melanin content of these hair follicles. Whether higher fluences or additional laser sessions would be more successful in treating lighter hair colours has yet to be determined.

Overall, the authors noted that patients with brown hair, skin phenotype III and lower extremity involvement responded best to treatment. This may suggest that there could be subgroups uniquely susceptible to laser hair removal. The authors also concurred that multiple sessions of treatment are required for optimal results.

# Jackson et al.[5]

Jackson et al. noted somewhat similar findings to those of Nanni and Alster. They evaluated 8 subjects with Fitzpatrick skin phenotypes III–IV. Subjects with unwanted hair on the legs, beard, bikini area, and axilla were treated with a 5 and 20ms alexandrite laser and fluences between 14 and 20J/cm². Both pulse durations led to equal hair removal efficacy. In addition, although there was histologic evidence of epidermal damage with both pulse durations, there was, as would be expected, less than 1 month of postinflammatory hyperpigmentation with the longer 20ms pulse duration.

The same authors then evaluated the effect of a 20ms and a 40ms alexandrite laser in individuals with similar complexions. Fifteen subjects were treated with fluences varying between 12 and 17J/cm². Although the clinical response was similar, there were greater pigmentary changes in the 20ms group compared with the 40ms group. In addition, the authors noted greater pain when the longer pulse duration was used.

# Rogers et al.[6]

Rogers et al. evaluated alexandrite laser hair removal in 15 subjects.[6] All were Fitzpatrick skin phenotypes I–III; all had blond or brown hair. Only axillae were treated. A 20ms alexandrite laser was utilized through a cooled gel. The laser was delivered with a 10–20% overlap, with a fluence of 22J/cm². The authors found that 80% of treated individuals had post-laser erythema, which lasted on average 2–3 days; 47% showed perifollicular erythema which lasted on average 90 hours. At 2 months, 55% of the hair was absent. However, at 3 months only 19% of the hair was absent. It should be noted that the findings might have been improved if only the darker hairs had been treated (D Glaser, personal communication). The findings of Rogers et al. are consistent with those of Nanni and Alster. An identical alexandrite laser was used in both studies. None of the subjects treated by Rogers et al. were noted to have pigmentary changes. Scarring also did not occur.

## Touma and Rohrer[7]

Touma and Rohrer evaluated a 3ms alexandrite laser, used in conjunction with −30°C cryogen spray cooling. They evaluated 21 subjects, 12–15 months after one treatment with average fluences of $33J/cm^2$. The presumed permanent hair reduction was noted to be 30% at this period. In addition, the authors noted a 29% reduction in the width of the remaining hairs.

## Avram[8]

In a somewhat similar study to that of Touma and Rohrer, Avram evaluated the same 3ms alexandrite laser, used in conjunction with −30°C cryogen spray cooling. Using a variety of fluences, he noted a 40–60% hair reduction after three treatments performed at 4–8 week intervals.[8] The follow-up intervals and treated anatomic sites varied in different individuals. Of great interest was the finding that 15% of treated individuals showed 80% hair reduction after three treatments and 15% of treated individuals showed less than 30% hair reduction after three treatments. This suggests that results can vary from individual to individual and from one anatomic region to the next. The findings are also consistent with anecdotal reports suggesting that there are rare individuals who, for unknown reasons, may not respond to laser hair removal.

The study also showed that both hyper- and hypopigmentation were more common in Fitzpatrick skin phenotypes IV–V. However, blisters and transient pigmentary changes were also observed in Fitzpatrick skin phenotype II–III individuals who had recent suntans.

Erythema, although universally present at the time of treatment, lasted between 12 and 48 hours in less than 5% of individuals.

## Goldberg and Akhami[9]

With R Akhami, I recently compared the effect of pulse duration and multiple treatments on alexandrite laser hair removal efficacy.[9] Fourteen subjects (3 men, 11 women) between the ages of 19 and 51 were studied. Treatment sites included the chin, neck, back, bikini area and lower leg; Fitzpatrick skin phenotypes were I–III. All subjects had black or brown terminal hairs.

An alexandrite laser with a pulse duration of 2ms, energy fluence of 25J/cm$^2$, 7mm spot size, and repetition rate of 5 pulses per second was compared with an alexandrite laser with a pulse duration of 10ms, energy fluence of 25J/cm$^2$, 7mm spot size, and a repetition rate of 3 pulses per second. A cooled gel was applied to the skin prior to treatment. Consecutive treatment and evaluations were made at 2- to 3-month intervals for a total of three treatment visits. Post-treatment complications such as erythema, pigmentary changes and scars were evaluated. The 2 and 10ms laser treatment results were compared, side by side, for a given anatomical site. Terminal hair counts were performed at baseline and compared with similar evaluations at 6 months following the final treatment. The percentage of hair loss was defined as the number of terminal hairs present after treatment compared with the number of terminal hairs present at baseline.

The average hair reduction was 33.1% for the 2ms pulse duration and 33.9% for the 10ms pulse duration. There was a slightly greater, albeit statistically insignificant, loss of thicker hairs (such as those seen on the back of men) with the 10ms alexandrite laser. The most common post-treatment complication was perifollicular erythema. This developed immediately after treatment and resolved within 24–48 hours. No cutaneous pigmentary changes or scarring was noted 6 months after the final treatment.

This study was unique, in that it was the first to compare two different pulse durations after multiple treatments. It should be noted that our results showed a greater degree of improvement than that seen in the studies of both Nanni and Alster and Rogers et al. This may be due to the higher number of treatment sessions or the slightly higher delivered fluences utilized in our study. We initially expected that the 10mn alexandrite laser would be more effective because of the greater confinement of thermal damage to the follicle. The purported benefit of this longer pulse duration may be equalled, though, by the greater peak power seen with a 2ms laser system. Although our study showed an overall reduction of hair counts, there was no significant difference between the different pulse durations. Despite this lack of clinical difference, the 2ms pulse duration laser may ultimately be the better practical treatment alternative, when all other chosen parameters are equal, because of its faster speed (5 pulses per second vs. 3 pulses per second). It should also be noted, though, that an even longer pulsed laser system might be safer in darker skin phenotypes not evaluated in this study.

# AVAILABLE ALEXANDRITE LASER SYSTEMS

## EpiTouch (ESC/Sharplan, Norwood, MA)

The EpiTouch is a normal mode alexandrite laser. This laser removes hair in a manner somewhat similar to that seen with ruby lasers. This system uses a cooling transparent gel to minimize reflectance and scattering. The cooling lessens thermal injury to the epidermis. A template is used to allow precise treatment of all hairs in

81

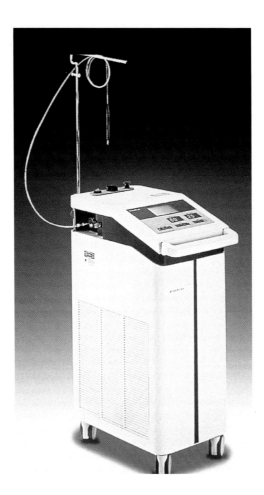

**Figure 5.4.** EpiTouch alexandrite laser

a particular area. The parameters for this system are 2–40ms emitted pulses at up to 5Hz with a 5–10mm beam diameter (Figure 5.4). The laser can be utilized with a scanner that allows a 50 × 50mm scan pattern. Fluences of up to 50J/cm² can be delivered with a treatment speed up to 240cm²/minute.

## GentleLASE (Candela Laser, Wayland, MA)

The GentleLASE is a normal mode alexandrite laser (Figure 5.5). This laser removes hair in a manner somewhat similar to that seen with ruby lasers. This system uses an integrated dynamic cooling device. The cryogen, delivered in adjustable spray durations of 20–100ms, lessens thermal injury to the epidermis. The laser delivers a 3ms pulse at 1Hz with 8, 10, 12, and 15mm beam diameters. Fluences of up to 100J/cm² can be delivered with the 8mm spot size; fluences up to 30J/cm² are obtainable with the 15mm spot size.

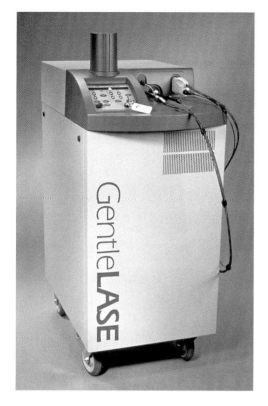

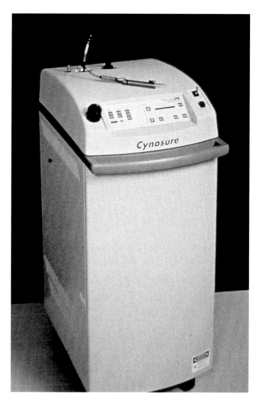

**Figure 5.5.** GentleLASE alexandrite laser

**Figure 5.6.** Apogee alexandrite laser

## LPIR and Apogee-40 (Cynosure, Chelmsford, MA)

The LPIR was the original alexandrite laser manufactured by Cynosure. The Apogee-40 is a newer more powerful alexandrite laser than is its predecessor (Figure 5.6). Pulse durations of 5, 10, 20, and 40ms can be delivered with up to a 12.5mm spot size; the newer Apogee system can deliver fluences of 5–40J/cm².

## MY APPROACH

I have found the alexandrite lasers to be very useful in treating Fitzpatrick I and II skin phenotypes. Although it has been suggested that alexandrite lasers, with a longer 755nm wavelength, are safer in treating darker complexions than are ruby lasers, I have not consistently found this to be the case. It would appear that the ability to treat darker complexions is more a factor of longer pulse durations (40ms with

EpiTouch and Apogee alexandrite lasers). Unless appropriate cooling is utilized, Fitzpatrick skin phenotype III and even sun-tanned type II complexioned individuals tend to have postinflammatory pigmentary changes.

Alexandrite laser speed is helped by the availability of scanning devices (EpiTouch) or large delivered spot sizes (Apogee or GentleLASE). Unlike the bulkiness of some ruby laser articulated delivery systems, alexandrite laser irradiation is delivered through lightweight fiber-optic systems.

The treatment technique commences with preoperative shaving of the treatment site. This reduces treatment-induced odor, prevents long pigmented hairs that lie on the skin surface from conducting thermal energy to the adjacent epidermis and promotes transmission of laser energy down the hair follicle. In darkly pigmented or heavily tanned individuals, it may be beneficial to use topical hydroquinones and meticulous sunscreen protection for several weeks prior to treatment in order to reduce inadvertent injury to epidermal pigment. Postinflammatory pigmentary changes still are to be expected in some individuals who have darker complexions.

The alexandrite laser, at almost all fluences, can lead to temporary hair loss in all treated areas. However, choosing appropriate anatomic locations, higher fluences, and treating hair multiple times will increase the likelihood of permanent hair reduction (Figures 5.7 to 5.43).

The ideal treatment parameters must be individualized for each patient, based on clinical experience and professional judgment. The novice may wish to deliver several individual test pulses at an inconspicuous site with equivalent pigmentation, starting

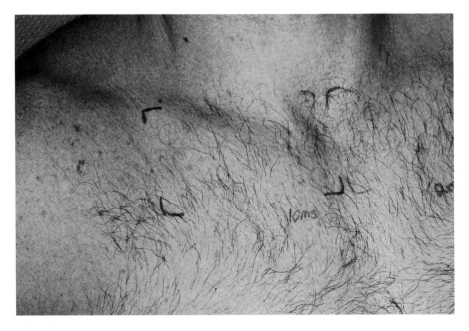

**Figure 5.7.** Upper chest before treatment with an alexandrite laser

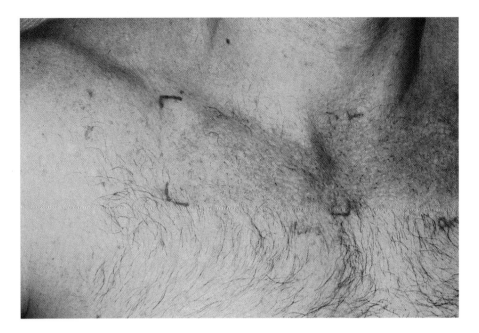

**Figure 5.8.** Expected erythema immediately after alexandrite laser treatment

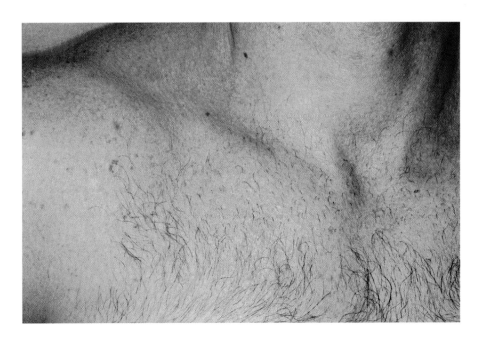

**Figure 5.9.** Beginning of hair regrowth 3 months after one alexandrite laser treatment

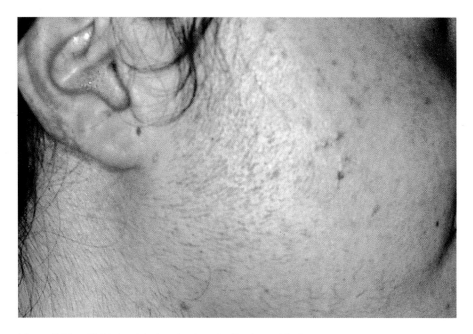

**Figure 5.10.** Right cheek before treatment with alexandrite laser

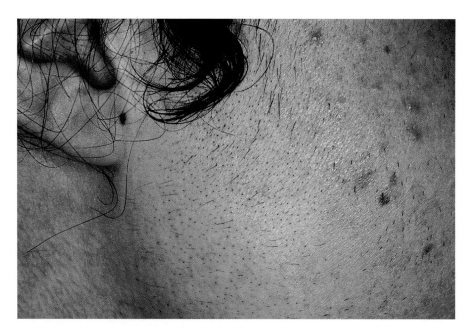

**Figure 5.11.** Right cheek 4 months after three alexandrite laser sessions. Note thinning of some hairs intermixed with areas of minimal regrowth

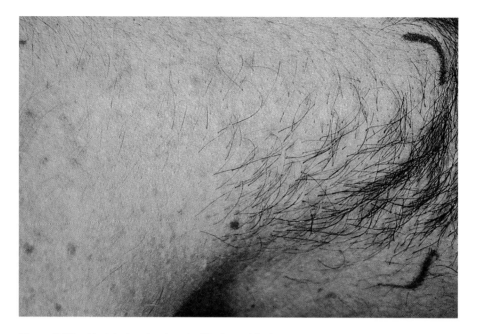

**Figure 5.12.** Neck before treatment with alexandrite laser treatment

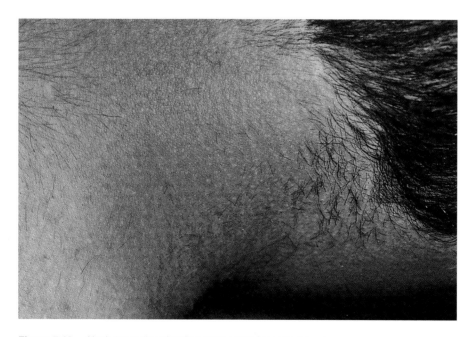

**Figure 5.13.** Neck 3 months after first alexandrite laser treatment

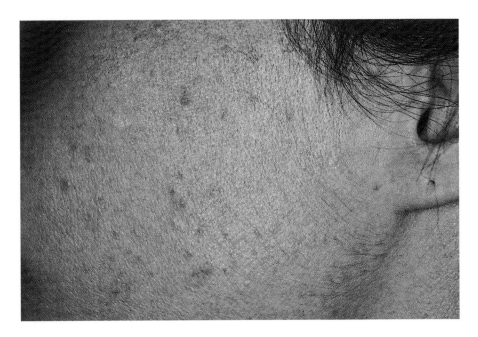

**Figure 5.14.** Left cheek before alexandrite laser treatment

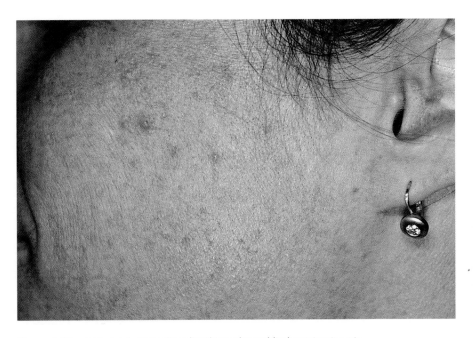

**Figure 5.15.** Left cheek 5 months after three alexandrite laser treatments

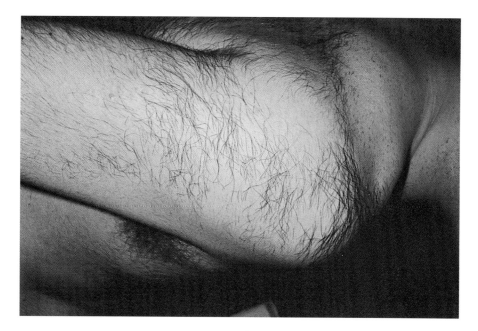

**Figure 5.16.** Right shoulder before alexandrite laser treatment

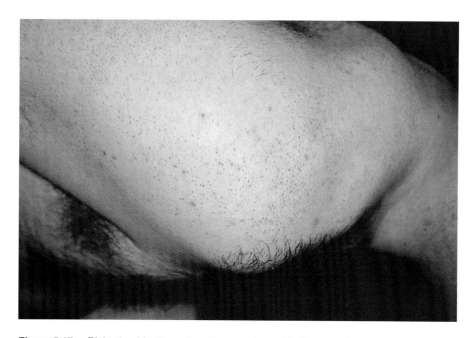

**Figure 5.17.** Right shoulder 2 months after one alexandrite laser treatment

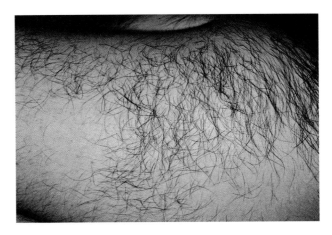

**Figure 5.18.** Left shoulder before alexandrite laser treatment

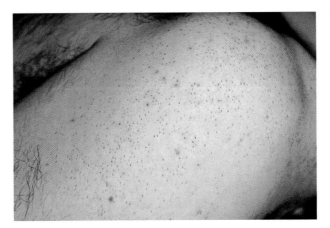

**Figure 5.19.** Left shoulder 1 month after one alexandrite laser treatment

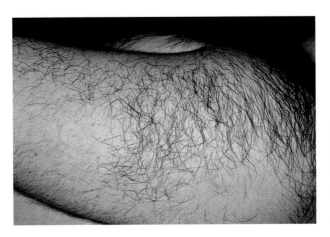

**Figure 5.20.** Left shoulder 4 months after one alexandrite laser treatment. Note that almost all hairs have regrown after only one session

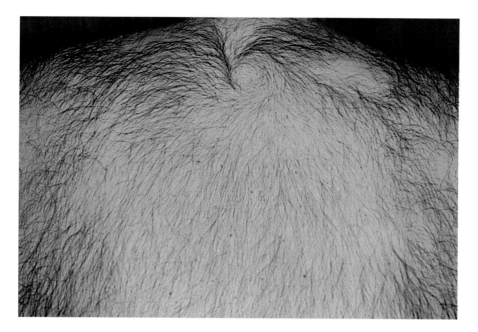

**Figure 5.21.** Back before alexandrite laser treatment

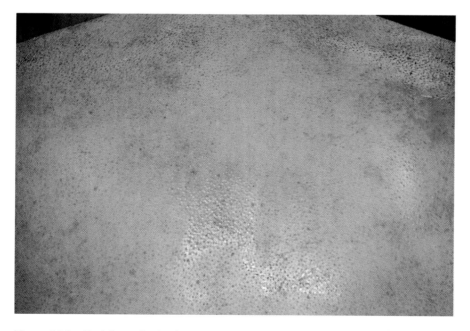

**Figure 5.22.** Back immediately after alexandrite laser treatment

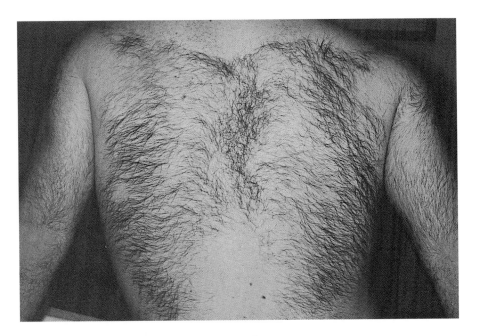

**Figure 5.23.** Back before alexandrite laser treatment

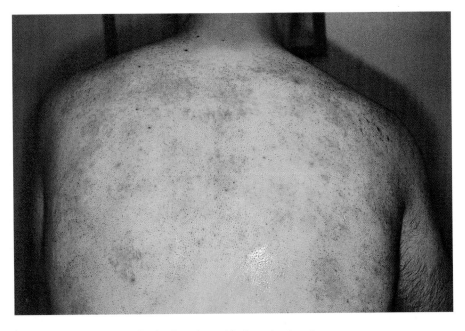

**Figure 5.24.** Back immediately after alexandrite laser treatment

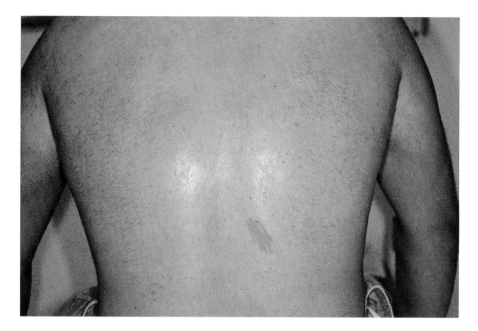

**Figure 5.25.** Back 3 months after one alexandrite laser treatment

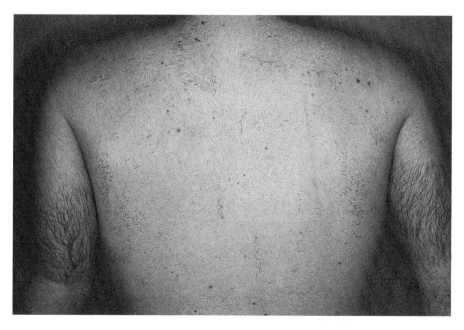

**Figure 5.26.** Back 4 months after third alexandrite laser treatment. Note some areas on upper back have regrown

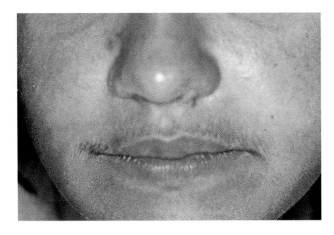

**Figure 5.27.** Upper lip in Fitzpatrick IV skin phenotype before alexandrite laser treatment

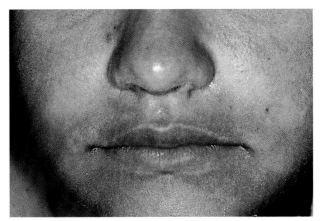

**Figure 5.28.** Upper lip in Fitzpatrick IV skin phenotype immediately after alexandrite laser treatment. Treatment was undertaken with extensive pretreatment cooling using GentleLASE laser cryogen-induced cooling. This lessened post-treatment epidermal blistering

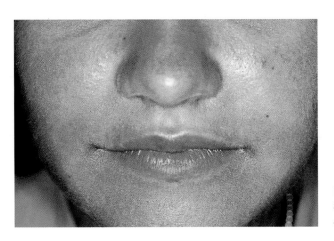

**Figure 5.29.** Upper lip 3 months after two alexandrite laser sessions

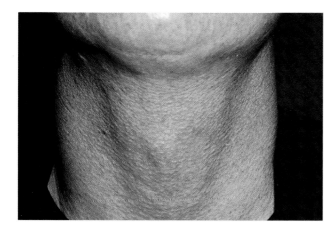

**Figure 5.30.** Neck before alexandrite laser treatment

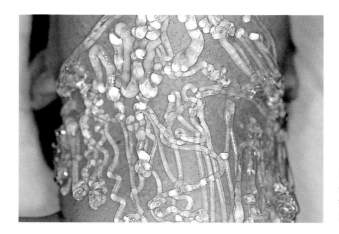

**Figure 5.31.** Cooling gel applied before use of the EpiTouch alexandrite laser

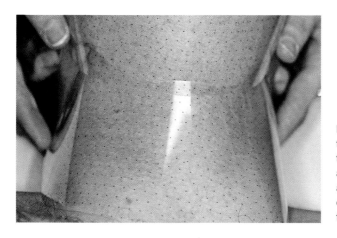

**Figure 5.32.** EpiTouch template being applied to the skin before alexandrite laser. This allows exact placement of each 7mm laser spot from this laser

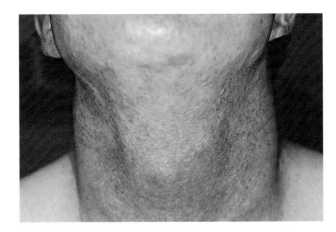

**Figure 5.33.** Expected erythema immediately after alexandrite laser treatment

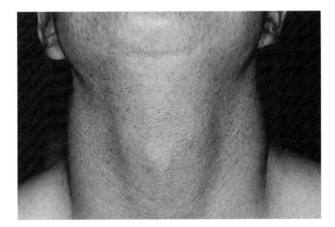

**Figure 5.34.** Neck 3 months after three alexandrite laser treatments

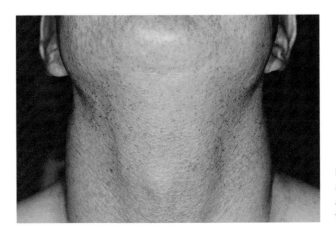

**Figure 5.35.** Neck 5 months after four alexandrite laser treatments

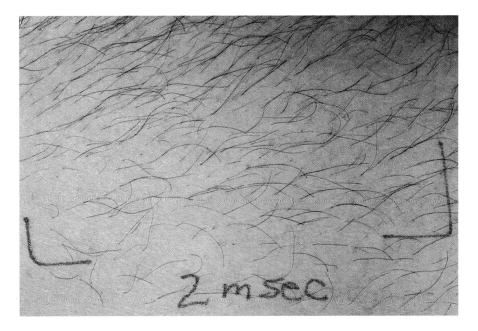

**Figure 5.36.**  Left bikini before alexandrite laser treatment

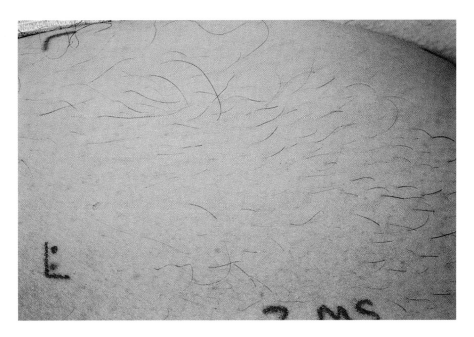

**Figure 5.37.**  Left bikini 6 months after three alexandrite laser treatments

**Figure 5.38.** Left bikini before alexandrite laser treatment

**Figure 5.39.** Left bikini 9 months after two alexandrite laser treatments

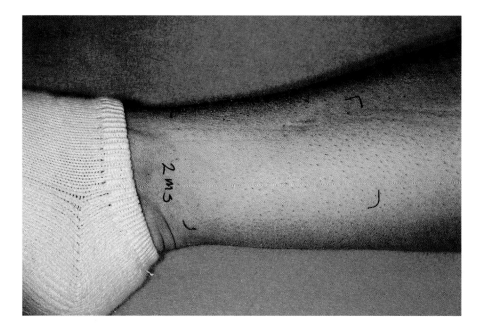

**Figure 5.40.** Left leg before alexandrite laser treatment

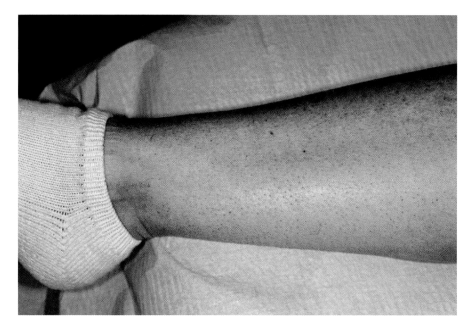

**Figure 5.41.** Left leg 2 months after alexandrite laser treatment

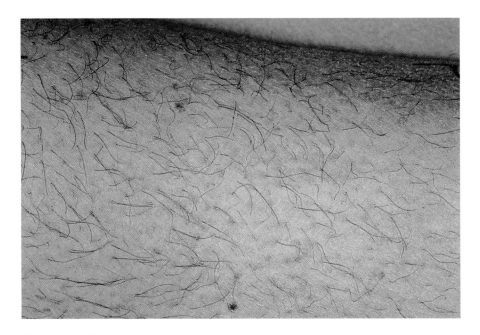

**Figure 5.42.**   Right leg before alexandrite laser treatment

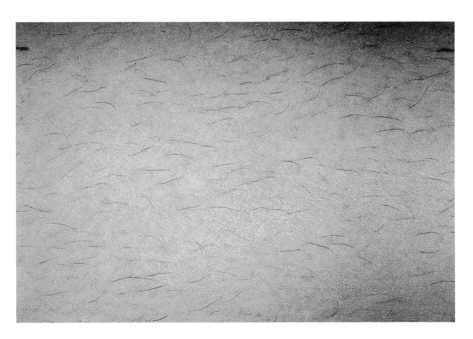

**Figure 5.43.**   Right leg 3 months after second alexandrite laser treatment

at an energy fluence of 15J/cm² and slowly increasing the delivered energy. As a general rule, somewhat lower fluences are required for effective hair removal than are required with ruby lasers. This may be related to the deeper penetration of the 755nm wavelength. Undesirable epidermal changes such as whitening and blistering are to be avoided.

Prolonged and permanent hair loss may occur following the use of all normal model alexandrite lasers; however, great variation in treatment results is often seen. Most patients with brown or black hair obtain a 2- to 6-month growth delay after a single treatment. There is usually only mild discomfort at the time of treatment. Pain may be diminished by the use of topical or injected anesthetics.

Transient erythema and edema are occasionally seen and irregular pigmentation of 1–3 months duration has also been described. No permanent skin change, depigmentation, or scarring has been reported in the literature. Nevertheless, scarring has been anecdotally reported and is always a possibility. Such findings are identical to those with the ruby lasers.

# REFERENCES

1  Finkel B, Eliezri YD, Waldman A, et al. Pulsed alexandrite laser technology for noninvasive hair removal. J Clin Laser Med Surg 1997;15:225–9.
2  Woo TY, Molnar G. Laser assisted hair removal using the Cynosure long pulse alexandrite laser. Lasers Surg Med 1998;18(Suppl 10):38.
3  Narukar V, Miller HM, and Seltzer R. The safety and efficacy of the long pulse alexandrite laser for hair removal in various skin types. Lasers Surg Med 1998;18(Suppl 10):38.
4  Nanni C, Alster TS. Long-pulsed alexandrite laser-assisted hair removal at 5, 10, and 20 millisecond pulse durations. Lasers Surg Med 1999;24:332–7.
5  Jackson BA, Junkins-Hopkins J. Effect of pulsewidth variation on hair removal in ethnic skin. Presented at American Society for Dermatologic Surgery Meeting, Miami Beach, USA, May 1999.
6  Rogers CJ, Glaser DA, Siegfried EC, Walsh PM. Hair removal using topical suspension-assisted Q-switched Nd:YAG and long-pulsed alexandrite lasers: a comparative study. Derm Surg 1999;11:844–50.
7  Touma DJ, Rohrer TE. The 3msec long pulse alexandrite laser for hair removal. Presented at American Society for Dermatologic Surgery Meeting, Miami Beach, USA, May 1999.
8  Avram M. Alexandrite laser hair removal. Presented at 8th International Symposium on Cosmetic Laser Surgery, New Orleans, USA, March 1999.
9  Goldberg, DJ, Akhami R. An evaluation comparing short and long pulsed durations using the alexandrite laser for noninvasite hair removal. Lasers Surg Med 1999;25:223–8.

# 6 DIODE LASER

## KEY POINTS

(1) Diode lasers emit 800nm near-infrared wavelength
(2) There is good melanin absorption, albeit less than that seen with ruby and alexandrite lasers
(3) The risk of post-treatment pigmentary changes is slightly less than with ruby and alexandrite lasers (risk is lessened if significant cooling is applied or when longer pulse durations are utilized)
(4) The 800nm wavelength penetrates deeper into dermis than 694nm and 755nm wavelengths
(5) Diode systems are the smallest laser hair removal systems available. As such, they are easily movable from room to room
(6) Millisecond high fluence systems have been cleared by the US FDA for permanent hair reduction

## BACKGROUND

Semiconductor diode lasers are among the most efficient light sources available. Because such lasers tend to be smaller than flashlamp devices, they are well suited for clinical applications. The ruby, alexandrite, Nd:YAG lasers and intense pulsed light sources are all flashlamp-type devices. Thus, diode technology does represent a change from all other currently available hair removal devices. The currently available diode systems emit 800nm pulsed light. The 800nm wavelength is not as well absorbed by melanin as the 694nm ruby and 755nm alexandrite wavelengths (Figure 6.1). Conversely, though, the longer 800nm wavelength penetrates deeper into the hair follicle with a correspondingly greater chance of injuring follicular growth centers.

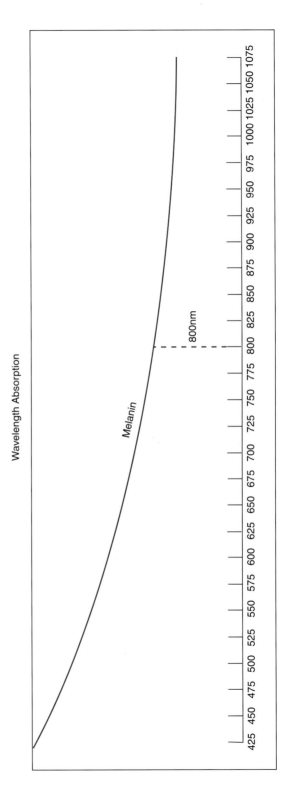

**Figure 6.1.** Melanin absorption curve of 800nm diode laser irradiation

# CLINICAL STUDIES

Diode lasers are among the newest of the available hair removal lasers. Dierickx et al.[1-3] have evaluated the effectiveness and safety of a pulsed diode laser in the permanent reduction of unwanted hair. Ninety-five subjects were evaluated. Different hair colors and skin types (Fitzpatrick skin types II–VI) were treated. The majority had Fitzpatrick II–III skin phenotypes and brown or black hair. Subjects were treated and examined at baseline, 1, 3, 6, 9, and 12 months after treatment. The objective of the study was not only to investigate effectiveness and safety of a pulsed diode laser in the permanent reduction of pigmented hair but also to study the fluence-responding relationship. The authors also evaluated one treatment versus two and single-pulse versus multiple-pulse treatments of the same area.

The device used by Dierickx et al. was a semiconductor diode laser system that delivers pulsed infrared light at a wavelength of 800nm, pulse duration of 5–20ms, and fluences from 15 to 40J/cm$^2$. In this particular study, the laser handpiece contained a high-power diode array, eliminating the need for an articulated arm or fiber-optic beam delivery system. Laser energy was delivered over a $9 \times 9$mm area. The handpiece contained an actively cooled convex sapphire lens that, when pressed against the subject's skin slightly before and during each laser pulse, provided thermal protection for the epidermis. The cooling lens was designed not only to allow higher doses of laser energy to target hair follicles safely and effectively but also to allow compression of the target area, placing hair roots closer to the laser energy.

The results demonstrated two different effects on hair growth: hair growth delay and permanent hair reduction. A measurable growth delay was seen in all patients (100%) at all fluence/pulse width configurations tested; this growth delay was sustained for 1–3 months.

Significant fluence-dependent, long-term hair reduction occurred in 88% of subjects. Clinically obvious long-term hair reduction usually required $\geqslant$30J/cm$^2$. After two treatments at 40J/cm$^2$ with a 20ms pulse duration, the average permanent hair reduction at the end of the study was 46%. Two treatments significantly increased hair reduction in comparison with one treatment, with an apparently additive effect. At a fluence of 40J/cm$^2$, the initial treatment removed approximately 30% of terminal hairs, and the second treatment given 1 month later removed an additional 25%. Triple pulsing of the same area did not significantly increase hair reduction over single pulsing, after one or two treatments. However, the incidence of side-effects was higher for triple pulsing.

It is noteworthy that hair regrowth stabilized at 6 months at all fluences; there was no further hair regrowth between 6-, 9-, and 12-months follow-up in this study. This stabilizing of hair regrowth or hair count is consistent with the generally accepted understanding of the growth cycle of many hair follicles. It is also consistent with the definition of permanent hair reduction – a significant reduction in the number of terminal hairs after treatment, which is stable for a longer period than the complete growth cycle of follicles at the body site tested.

In addition to statistically significant hair reduction, treatment also showed reduction in hair diameter and reduction in color of regrowing hairs. The mean regrown hair diameter decreased by 19.9% of baseline. Optical transmission at 700nm of hair shafts regrown post-treatment was 1.4 times greater than transmission pretreatment. Put differently, the hairs remaining after treatment were lighter and thinner.

Histologic analysis suggested that there are two mechanisms for effective, permanent reduction of terminal hair: miniaturization of coarse hair follicles to become vellus-like hair follicles; and destruction of the follicle, with granulomatous degeneration with a fibrotic remnant. Immediately after treatment, hairs in follicles with large pigmented shafts showed evidence of thermal damage. Follicles that had small vellus shafts showed no effect. Both pigmented and non-pigmented areas of terminal hair follicle epithelium showed thermal coagulation necrosis, with minimal or no damage to the adjacent dermis. Triple pulsing did not produce more follicular damage than single pulsing, although triple pulsing occasionally injured the dermis between closely spaced follicles. Sebaceous glands near the treated follicles showed no or minimal thermal damage. Sweat glands and dermal capillaries appeared normal.

As would be expected from any melanin-absorbing system, side-effects with pulsed diode laser treatment were fluence- and skin type-dependent. Hyper- or hypopigmentation was minimal in fair skin, and increased with fluence and with darker skin type. At the highest delivered fluence of $40J/cm^2$, the incidence of hyper- or hypopigmentation was greater for patients with skin types III to VI. In addition, clinical experience has shown that these high fluences may elicit somewhat greater side-effects in treatments of areas of high hair density.

The typical response of perifollicular erythema and edema was noted. Approximately 20% of patients exhibited pigment changes, which resolved in 1–3 months. The vast majority of pigment changes were transient, but with darker skin types and higher fluences, some persistent pigment changes were noted. Triple pulsing, as mentioned earlier, increased the incidence of hyper- or hypopigmentation compared with single pulsing, but did not significantly increase hair reduction.

It should be noted that in this study, all subjects with all skin types were treated with both low and high fluences. In clinical practice, fluence and pulse width can be adjusted for skin types. When this is done, the incidence of side-effects would be expected to be very small.

Adrian has noted that most patients experience more than 60% of long-term clearance (greater than 6 months) after two or three treatments (R Adrian, personal communication). Postoperative complications observed by him were limited to epidermal crusting and temporary hypopigmentation in darker skin type patients. He noted, as would be expected, that fair-skinned dark-haired subjects experienced excellent results; however, even skin type V patients could be treated safely with a longer (30ms) pulse duration, effective cooling, and slightly lesser fluences. Although no evidence of persistent pigmentary changes or textural changes were noted, the possibility of such complications from any laser or light source for hair removal must be considered.

# AVAILABLE DIODE LASER SYSTEMS

## LightSheer EP (Coherent Medical, Santa Clara, CA)

The LightSheer EP is the second-generation diode laser from the Coherent company (Figure 6.2). The laser is an 800nm near-infrared system with delivered fluences varying between 10 and 60J/cm$^2$. The machine delivers a pulse between 5 and 20ms and a longer 30ms pulse for darker complected individuals. The spot size is $9 \times 9$mm and cooling is of the 0°C contact-cooling type. The difference between the newer EP version and its predecessor lies in the higher delivered fluences (60 vs. 40J/cm$^2$) and faster speed (2 vs. 1Hz).

## LaserLite (Diomed, Cambridge, UK)

The LaserLite is a quasi-continuous wave 800nm diode laser that utilizes a scanning delivery system. Pulse durations are 50–250ms with 2 and 4mm spot sizes and contact cooling (Figure 6.3).

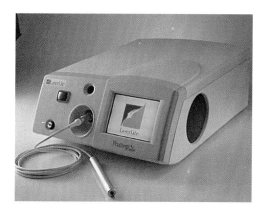

**Figure 6.3.** LaserLite laser

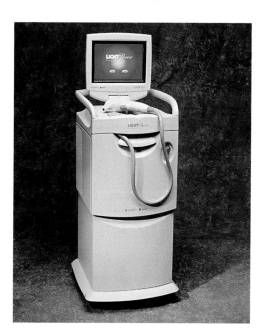

**Figure 6.2.** LightSheer EP laser

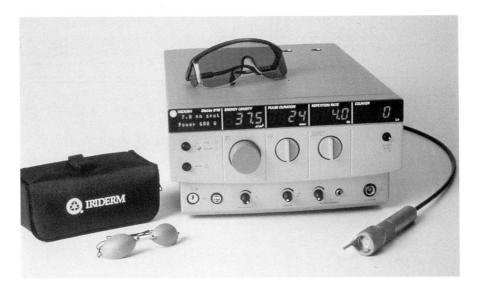

**Figure 6.4.** Iriderm-800 laser

## EpiStar (Nidek)

The EpiStar is a quasi-continuous wave 800nm diode laser with pulse durations up to 100ms, fluences up to 50J/cm², and 4 and 7mm spot sizes.

## Iriderm-800 (Iris Medical, Mountain View, CA)

This diode laser delivers fluences up to 40J/cm² with pulse durations varying between 10 and 30ms through a 7–10mm spot size. This quasi-continuous wave 800nm diode laser utilizes contact cooling (Figure 6.4).

## MY APPROACH

I have found the diode laser (LightSheer) very useful in treating Fitzpatrick I and IV skin phenotypes. The laser should always be used with the contact-cooling device. When used with the longer 30ms pulse duration, Fitzpatrick skin phenotypes can be treated with a lessening of postinflammatory pigmentary changes. Diode systems are small, portable and very user-friendly.

The treatment technique commences with preoperative shaving of the treatment site. This reduces treatment-induced odor, prevents long pigmented hairs that lie on the skin surface from conducting thermal energy to the adjacent epidermis, and promotes transmission of laser energy down the hair follicle. In darkly pigmented or heavily tanned individuals, it may be beneficial to use topical hydroquinones and meticulous sunscreen protection for several weeks prior to treatment in order to reduce inadvertent injury to epidermal pigment. Postinflammatory pigmentary changes still are to be expected in some individuals who have darker complexions. Transient perifollicular erythema and edema are also to be expected (Figure 6.5). Such findings are identical to those with the ruby and alexandrite lasers.

The diode laser, when used at almost all fluences, can lead to temporary hair loss at all treated areas. However, choosing appropriate anatomic locations, higher fluences, and treating hair multiple times will increase the likelihood of permanent hair reduction. (Figures 6.5 to 6.42).

As a consequence, the ideal treatment parameters must be individualized for each patient, based on clinical experience and professional judgment. The novice may choose to deliver several individual test pulses at an inconspicuous site with equivalent pigmentation, starting at an energy fluence of $20J/cm^2$ and slowly increasing the energy. As a general rule, somewhat lower fluences are required for effective hair removal than are required with the ruby lasers. This may be related to the deeper penetration of the 800nm wavelength. Undesirable epidermal changes such as whitening and blistering are to be avoided. There are no reports of scarring thus far. However, it is unrealistic to assume that this cannot occur.

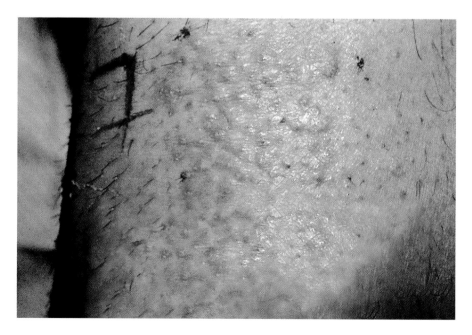

**Figure 6.5.** Perifollicular erythema seen immediately after LightSheer diode laser treatment. (Photo courtesy of M Grossman, MD.)

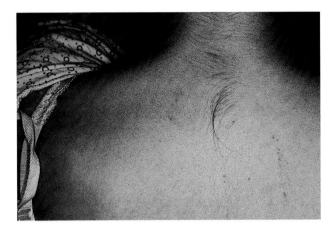

**Figure 6.6.** Dark neck hairs before treatment with the diode laser

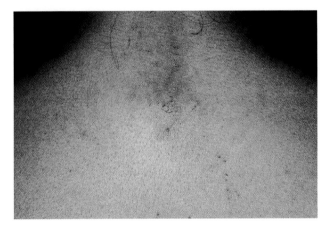

**Figure 6.7.** Expected erythema seen immediately after treatment

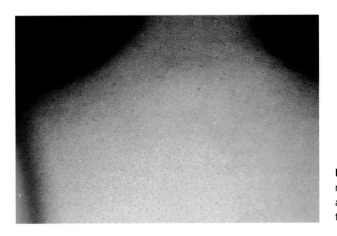

**Figure 6.8.** Absence of neck hairs seen 5 months after two treatments with the diode laser

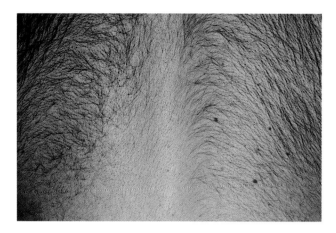

**Figure 6.9.** Male back hairs before treatment with the diode laser

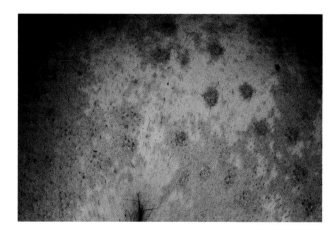

**Figure 6.10.** Immediately post-treatment

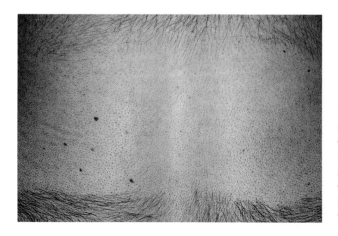

**Figure 6.11.** Upper back 4 months after one treatment with the diode laser, Mid-back 2 months after one treatment with the diode laser; the lower back has yet to be treated

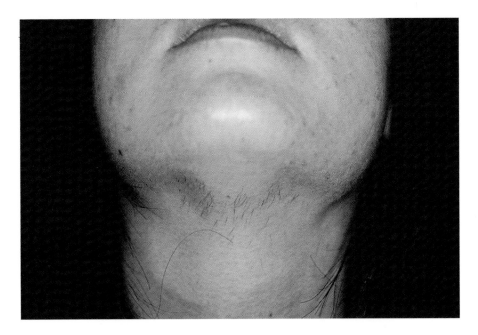

**Figure 6.12.** Hirsute chin prior to treatment with diode laser

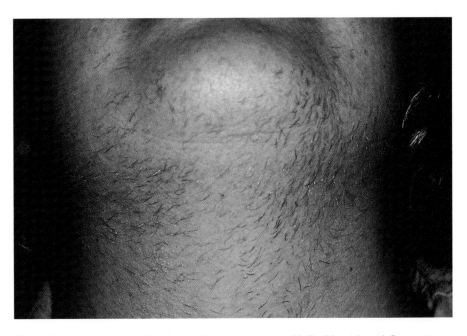

**Figure 6.13.** Close-up of chin. Note both hairs, presence of folliculitis and postinflammatory changes second to chronic inflammation

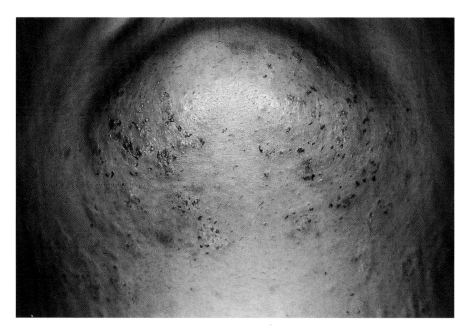

**Figure 6.14.** Immediately after treatment. Note the desired perifollicular erythema and edema

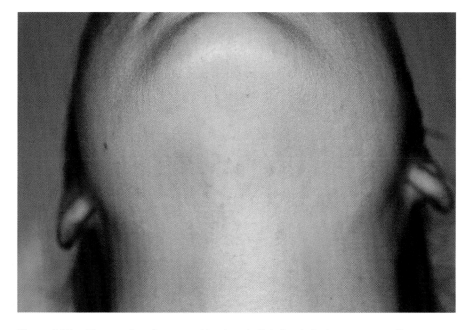

**Figure 6.15.** Five months after second treatment. Only fine hairs have regrown. Some postinflammatory hyperpigmentation persists

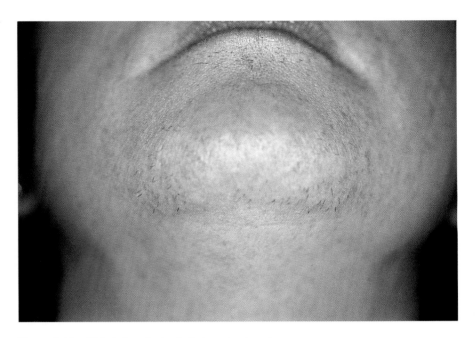

**Figure 6.16.** Chin hairs prior to diode laser treatment

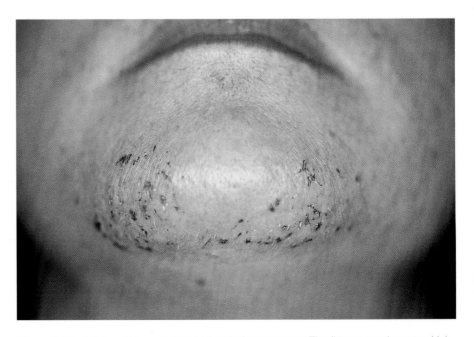

**Figure 6.17.** Mild crusting occasionally noted after treatment. The fluence used was too high

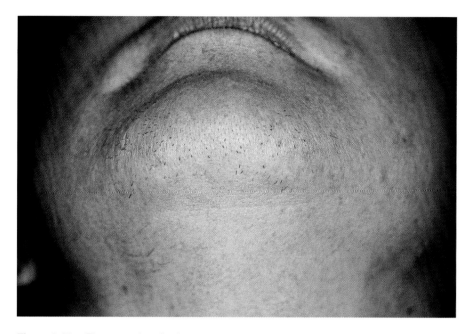

**Figure 6.18.** Three months after laser treatment. Note some improvement

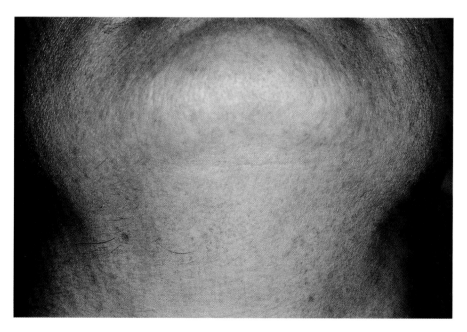

**Figure 6.19.** Six months after three sessions with the diode laser. Almost no hair has recurred

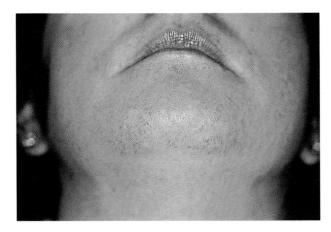

**Figure 6.20.** Chin hairs prior to treatment with the diode laser

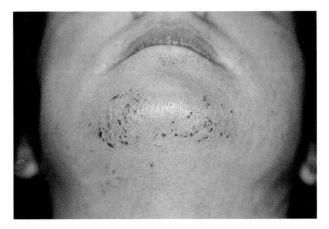

**Figure 6.21.** Perifollicular erythema and edema noted immediately after treatment

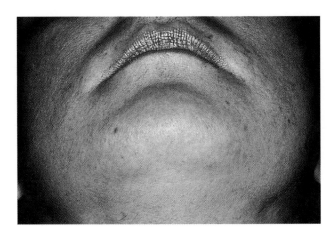

**Figure 6.22.** Six months after two sessions of diode laser treatment. Only several fine hairs have regrown

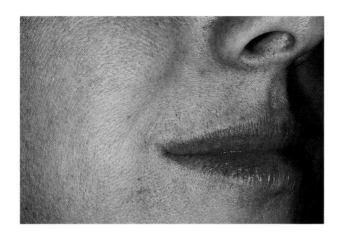

**Figure 6.23.** Fine upper lip hairs before treatment with the diode laser

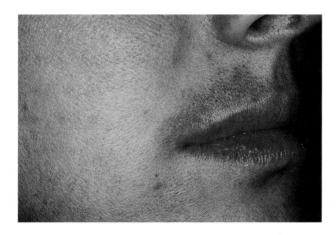

**Figure 6.24.** Erythema after diode laser treatment

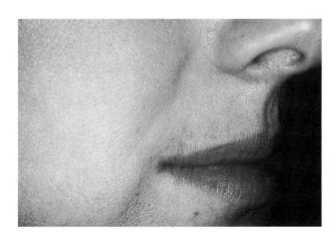

**Figure 6.25.** Three months after one session with the diode laser. All hairs have regrown. More sessions are required

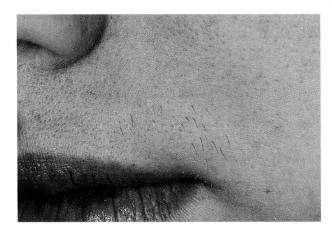

**Figure 6.26.** Fine upper lip hairs before treatment with the diode laser

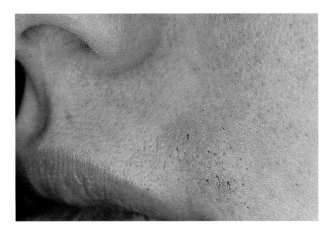

**Figure 6.27.** Mild erythema after the laser treatment

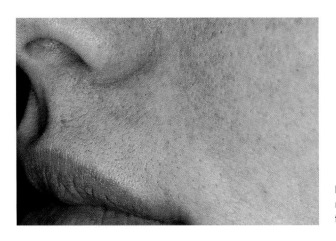

**Figure 6.28.** No regrowth 6 months after four diode laser sessions

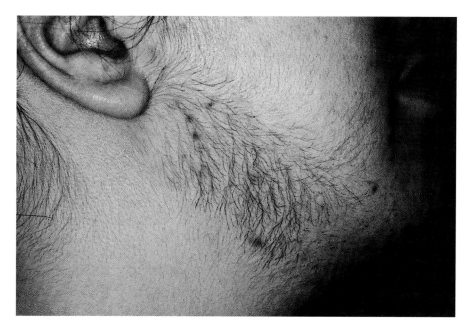

**Figure 6.29.** Right cheek hairs and folliculitis in patient with polycystic ovary disease. Treatment with spironolactone orally and seven sessions of electrolysis had minimal impact on hair growth

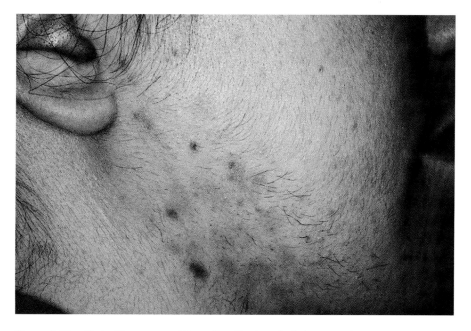

**Figure 6.30.** Marked improvement 5 months after four diode laser sessions

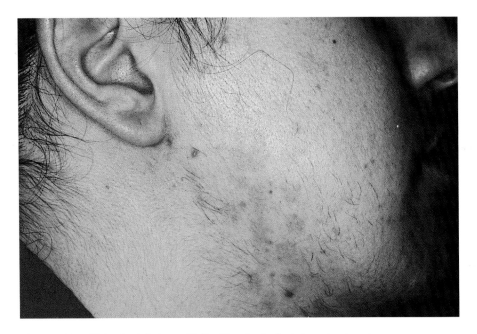

**Figure 6.31.** Right cheek hairs and folliculitis prior to diode laser treatment

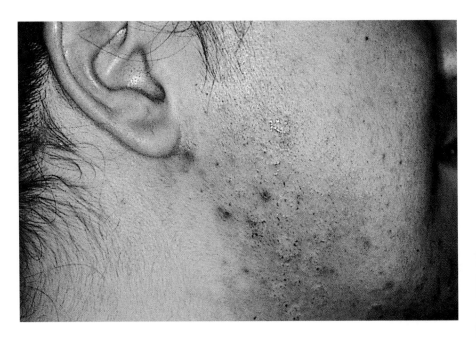

**Figure 6.32.** Erythema after laser treatment

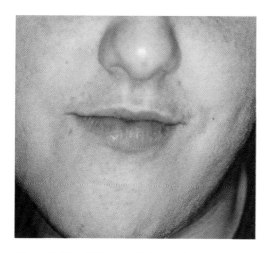

**Figure 6.33.** Mild upper lip hairs prior to diode laser treatment

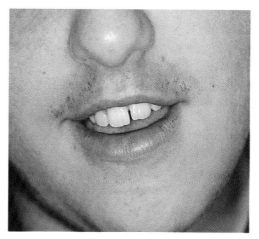

**Figure 6.34.** Expected erythema seen immediately after diode laser treatment

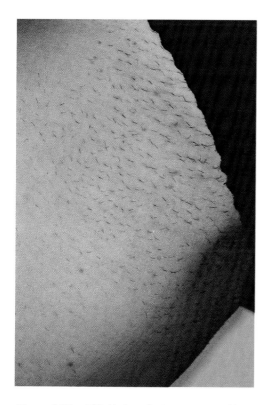

**Figure 6.35.** Bikini hairs prior to treatment with the diode laser

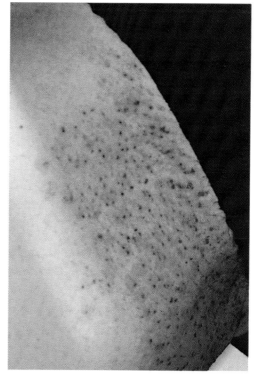

**Figure 6.36.** Expected perifollicular erythema and edema seen immediately after diode laser treatment

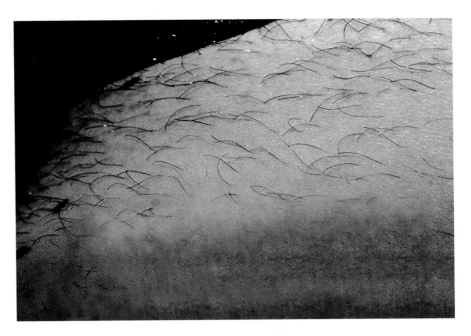

**Figure 6.37.** Bikini hairs prior to treatment with the LightSheer diode laser (Photo courtesy of M Grossman, MD.)

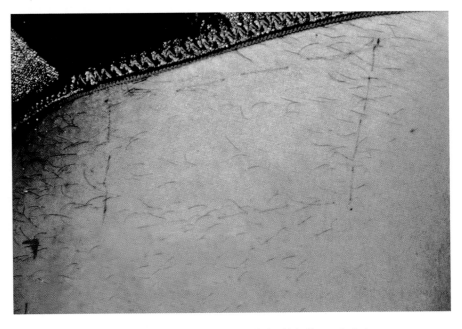

**Figure 6.38.** Bikini 5 months after one session with the LightSheer diode laser (Photo courtesy of M Grossman, MD.)

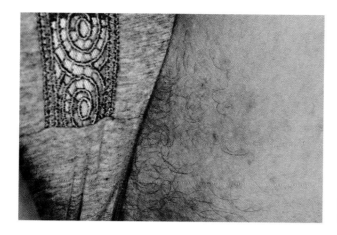

**Figure 6.39.** Bikini hairs prior to treatment with the diode laser

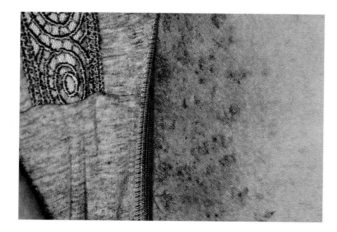

**Figure 6.40.** Expected erythema seen immediately after diode laser treatment

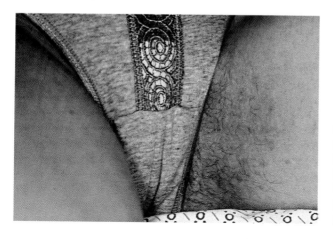

**Figure 6.41.** Bikini 6 months after two sessions with the diode laser. Some hairs have regrown. Hyperpigmentation present before treatment persists

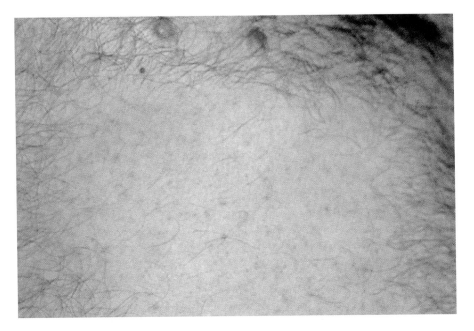

**Figure 6.42.** Absence of hair regrowth 1 year after Lightsheer diode laser treatment. Hypertropic scars are biopsy sites (Photo courtesy of M Grossman, MD.)

Prolonged and permanent hair loss may occur following the use of the diode laser. Most patients with brown or black hair obtain a 2- to 6-month growth delay after a single treatment. Long-term hair reduction can be expected as a result of multiple treatment sessions if appropriate fluences are utilized. There is usually only mild discomfort at the time of treatment. Pain may be diminished by the use of topical or injected anesthetics.

# REFERENCES

1   Dierickx CC, Grossman MC, Farinelli BS, et al. Hair removal by pulsed infrared diode laser. Lasers Surg Med 1998;10 (suppl):42.
2   Dierickx CC, Grossman MC, Farinelli BS, et al. Comparison between a long pulsed ruby laser and a pulsed infrared laser system for hair removal. Lasers Surg Med 1998;10 (suppl):42.
3   Grossman MC, Dierickx CC, Quintana A, et al. Removal of excess body hair with an 800nm pulsed diode laser. Lasers Surg Med 1998;10 (suppl):42.

# 7 Nd:YAG LASER

## KEY POINTS

(1) Nd:YAG lasers emit 1064nm infrared wavelength
(2) There is much less melanin absorption than with visible light wavelengths
(3) The risk of post-inflammatory pigmentary changes is significantly less than with visible light
(4) Penetration into the dermis is deeper than it is for visible light wavelengths
(5) Nanosecond pulse duration systems lead to only temporary hair reduction; newer millisecond pulse duration systems may lead to better results

## BACKGROUND

The Q-switched Nd:YAG laser emits a 1064nm wavelength beam with a pulse duration of 10 ns. Melanin is not a good absorbing chromophore of the 1064nm wavelength (Figure 7.1). Thus, 1064nm Q-switched Nd:YAG lasers have never been ideal for the treatment of benign pigmented lesions. Despite less melanin absorption of the 1064nm wavelength, compared with the wavelengths of ruby, alexandrite, and diode laser systems, the Nd:YAG laser's advantage lies in its ability to penetrate more deeply in the skin (up to 4–6mm). The nanosecond Q-switched Nd-YAG laser's effect on hair is one of photomechanical damage. In order to induce a photothermal effect on treated hairs, a millisecond Nd:YAG laser must be used.

In order to cause selective hair damage, an innate and unique property of the follicle must be attacked. Although melanin is the chromophore exploited most, other proteins could theoretically be targeted. Alternatively, an agent capable of laser absorption may be placed in proximity to the hair. If an appropriate topical chromophore is applied, penetrates around the hair, and is then activated by laser light, heating of this chromophore would in turn heat and damage the surrounding

126

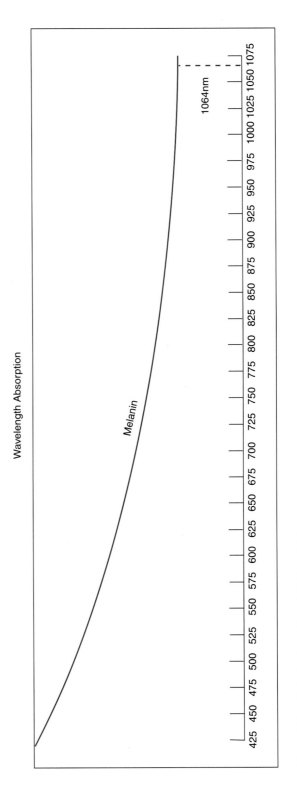

**Figure 7.1.** Melanin absorption of 1064nm light

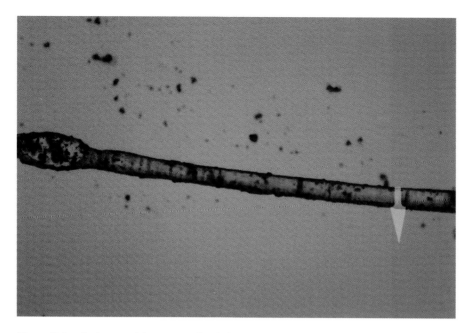

**Figure 7.2.** Carbon particles surrounding hair

follicle. In one of the first available laser hair removal methods, this technique was used. A Q-switched Nd:YAG laser was utilized in conjunction with a topical carbon-based suspension in an attempt to target, damage, and decrease unwanted hair (Figure 7.2).

# CLINICAL STUDIES

## Goldberg et al.[1–3]

In one of the first laser hair removal studies, 35 subjects (6 men, 29 women), ranging in age from 20 to 74 years, were treated.[1,2] Treatment sites included the upper lip, chin, cheeks, neck, and axillae. The hair was trimmed to a length of 1–2mm. A topical carbon/mineral oil suspension was then massaged into the treatment sites and allowed to absorb for 5–10 minutes. The excess suspension was then wiped away and was followed by laser treatment with a 1064nm Q-switched Nd:YAG laser. Laser energy was delivered with a 7mm diameter spot, a fluence of 2–3 J/cm$^2$, and a 10ns pulse. Patients were assessed at 4 and 12 weeks.

At week 4, the investigators evaluated 68 sites on the 35 treated subjects. Ten per cent of the sites showed 0–25% reduction in hair; 44% showed 26–50% reduction in hair; 24% showed 51–75% reduction in hair; and 22% showed 76–100% reduction in hair. By 3 months, the degree of hair reduction had decreased. At week 12, evaluation of 55 treated sites showed 27% with 0–25% clearance, 42% with 26–50% clearance, 12% with 51–75% clearance, and 18% with 76–100% clearance. In evaluating the data in a different manner, the authors noted greater than 25% hair reduction in 90% of subjects at week 4 and greater than 25% hair reduction in 73% of the subjects at week 12.

The only common reaction was erythema, seen immediate following treatment. Erythema resolved in all patients within 4–8 hours. One patient had mild hyperpigmentation, which had completely resolved at week 12. No patients showed any scars or texture changes.

It has been postulated that laser hair removal that is assisted by use of a topical carbon solution damages hair follicles in the following manner. Nd:YAG laser light is strongly absorbed by carbon (in contrast to other cutanous chromophores such as melanin). As the topical carbon interacts with 1064nm laser light, it undergoes a rapid temperature rise. The resulting photomechanical shock waves propel carbon particles in multiple directions. It is assumed that this effect, in some way, causes follicular damage with resultant delayed hair growth.

Goldberg et al.[1,2] suggested a potential melanin-sparing advantage in using a Nd:YAG laser system. Although the melanin-specific lasers are very useful for dark-haired individuals, patients with lighter or white hair respond poorly. The authors assumed that the presence of an exogenous chromophore coating these non-pigmented hairs would lead to better results. Furthermore, the longer 1064nm near-infrared wavelength leads to greater depth of follicular penetration, with the potential for greater follicular damage. Finally, because of the relative melanin-sparing capacity of 1064nm Nd:YAG laser energy, darker Fitzpatrick skin phenotypes (IV–VI) might be successfully treated.

It should be noted that, in comparison with the typical energy densities required in Q-switched Nd:YAG laser tattoo removal, fluences used in this study were very low. Less energy often translated into less pain. Even though this carbon assisted laser hair removal is not devoid of discomfort, most patients easily tolerate it. No patient in this study required a topical or local anesthetic. In addition, a lower fluence decreased the risk of adverse events. Permanent pigmentary changes were not seen in this study.

In a follow-up study, the results of a single treatment using a topical carbon suspension and Q-switched Nd:YAG laser were compared with the results seen after three treatments.[3] The parameters were similar to those used in the first study. Twelve female subjects with unwanted bikini and axillary hair were treated three times. The study revealed that cumulative treatments led to better results.

It should be noted that all treated individuals in both these studies had 1–2mm hairs at the time of treatment. In a variation on the technique utilized in these studies, hair has been waxed prior to the laser procedure. This was done in an attempt to allow greater carbon access to the deeper follicular structures. There has been no scientific evidence that this technique leads to better results.

# Nanni and Alster[4]

In a subsequent study, Nanni and Alster evaluated the effectiveness of topical carbon suspension assisted Q-switched Nd:YAG laser hair removal under varying pre-treatment protocols.[4] Laser hair removal was performed under four different pre-treatment conditions. Eighteen areas of unwanted body and facial hair from 12 study subjects were divided into four quadrants. Wax epilation followed by application of a carbon-based solution and exposure to Q-switched Nd:YAG laser radiation was performed on one quadrant. A second quadrant was wax epilated and exposed to Q-switched Nd:YAG laser radiation without prior carbon solution application. A third quadrant was exposed to laser radiation alone. A final quadrant was wax epilated to serve as the control. Follow-up evaluations were made at 1, 3, and 6-month intervals. The 12 subjects (3 men, 9 women) had a mean age of 32 years. The total of 18 anatomic sites included 6 backs, 3 upper lips, 1 chin, and 8 legs. Treated skin types included Fitzpatrick skin phenotypes I–IV. Only subjects with black or brown terminal hair were included in the study. A 1064nm Q-switched Nd:YAG laser was used at a fluence of 2.6J/cm$^2$, pulse duration of 50ns, and a 7mm spot size.

Follow-up evaluations consisted of manual hair counts and subjective hair-density estimates. The mean regrowth at 1 month was 39.9% for the wax–carbon–laser quadrants, 46.7% for the wax–laser quadrants, 66.1% for the laser-alone quadrants, and 77.9% for the wax control quadrants. At the 3-month follow-up, all laser-treated quadrants had significantly less hair regrowth than the control quadrant, with a mean regrowth of 79.1% for the wax–carbon–laser quadrants, 85.2% for the wax–laser quadrants, 86.3% for the laser-alone quadrants, and full regrowth for the wax control quadrants. All hair regrew in all quadrants by 6 months.

Subjective hair density estimates reflected the objective hair count data. It should be noted that several subjects did note changes in their hair quality after laser treatment. The regrown hairs were finer in texture and lighter in color. Such an observation is consistent with the theory that laser-induced damage occurs in both the growth center and the pigment production sites of treated hairs.

The results of this study suggested that after a single Q-switched Nd:YAG laser treatment, a change within the hair follicle is produced that results in a delay in hair regrowth. However, permanent hair reduction, the authors noted, was not achieved. The authors also found that although pre-treatment with wax epilation and topical carbon suspension results in significant hair removal, these protocols were not essential. All laser treated sites showed less hair regrowth at 3 months than the wax-epilated control sites. This suggested that the laser energy could be targeted in the follicle without an exogenous carbon chromophore. The authors were unable to determine the optimal pre-treatment protocol. They did suggest that when treating areas bearing blond or white hair, exogenous carbon application might lead to better results.

## McDaniel (unpublished)

In a recent study, McDaniel evaluated the use of a 5ns Q-switched Nd:YAG laser, without an exogenous carbon chromophore, for temporary hair removal (D McDaniel, personal communication). He found that at 2J/cm² there was little histologic damage to the dermis surrounding the treated hair follicle. In contrast there was obvious histologic damage to the hair shaft and follicular matrix. He noted that although 1064nm laser irradiation is not absorbed by melanin as well as are visible light wavelengths, the immediate whitening of treated hairs may reflect hair-shaft melanosome destruction. The study suggested that the depilatory effect of a low fluence, nanosecond, photomechanical laser system is one of growth delay. There appears to be premature telogen induction, rather than true photothermal damage to the hair structure.

## Bencini et al.[5]

Bencini et al. were the first to evaluate hair removal efficacy with a long-pulse millisecond Nd:YAG laser.[5] Such a system theoretically combines the pigmentation safety of a near-infrared laser with the photothermal benefits of millisecond pulsed technology.

Two hundred and eight subjects were treated during an 11-month period. The subjects were divided into three groups. Group A consisted of 79 subjects (8 men, 71 women); this group included subjects with normal size and distribution of hairs. Group B contained 67 subjects, all women, with constitutional familial hypertrichosis. Group C contained 62 patients (51 women, 11 transsexuals) with hirsutism. Most of the females in this third group had polycystic ovary syndrome. Subjects ranged in age from 18 to 56. Treated areas included the face and neck (30%), bikini area (27%), lip (22%), abdomen (13%), legs (14%), chin (12%), arms (5%), and axillae (3%). Two hundred and three subjects were Fitzpatrick skin phenotypes II–IV and 5 were Fitzpatrick skin phenotype V. Hair colors were divided as follows: 124 subjects with dark hair, 2 with white hair, 78 with blond hair, and 4 with red hair.

The number of treatment sessions was determined solely by the subject's desire to achieve aesthetic and psychological satisfaction with the results. The goal of treatment was not necessary to obtain complete epilation in all subjects. Thus, some subjects were treated only once, others many times.

The laser treatment was performed with a long-pulsed Nd:YAG laser. Laser energy was delivered at 3 or 4mm spot sizes and fluences between 23 and 56J/cm², depending on hair type. As a general rule, lower fluences were used for darker or finer hairs and higher fluences for lighter or thicker hairs.

The first session resulted in a 20–40% hair loss of the treated area, lasting over 24 weeks. These results were considered satisfactory by 21/79 patients who had the normal hair and normal anatomical distribution (Group A). Results were deemed satisfactory by all 67 patients of the constitutional hypertrichosis (Group B). It should be noted that these individuals often sought only improvement and not complete epilation. Group C patients and 58/79 of the patients in group A usually desired a greater degree of epilation. Thus, after 4 weeks they had a second treatment, with an incremental increase of 20–40% more hair loss. The authors noted a greater degree of improvement at higher fluences (40–56J/cm² compared with 30–40J/cm²). Higher fluences, however, also caused more discomfort. This led the subjects to often choose comfort over greater efficacy in their treatments. Surprisingly, the authors noted a good response in blond hair at all fluences used. Red hair also responded to laser treatment. White hair, as expected, did not respond to laser treatment. Biopsies from specimens obtains 6 hours after treatment revealed extensive necrosis of the hair follicle and sebaceous gland epithelium. Histologic findings in biopsies taken 3 months after the end of the treatment showed complete disappearance of hair follicles, with the occasional presence of arrector pili muscle and scattered focal fibrosis.

No patient showed any long-term pigmentary changes. This was significant in view of the fact that 5 treated subjects had Fitzpatrick V skin phenotypes. Mild transient erythema was present in all patients after the treatment sessions. This generally regressed within 1 to 2 hours after treatment. Of note was the fact that no blistering was noted at any fluence, even in Fitzpatrick IV–V skin phenotypes.

The authors suggested that long pulsed Nd:YAG treatment produces effective prolonged epilation after several sessions, with no significant side-effects. Unfortunately, nowhere in the article do they describe the pulse duration of the long-pulse Nd:YAG laser they used. It is noteworthy that the authors did suggest that with the 1064nm wavelength, other chromophores besides melanin (hemoglobin) may be absorbing laser energy.

# Goldberg[6]

In my own recent study, millisecond Nd:YAG laser treatment was performed on 15 healthy adult volunteers, ranging in age from 28 to 69 years.[6] Subjects were divided into two treatment groups: females with facial hair (group I), and females or males with non-facial hair (group II). Treatment sites included periorbital area (4 sites), cheeks (2 sites), sideburns (2 sites), bikini area (10 sites), back (6 sites), chest (3 sites), abdomen (1 site), and arms (1 site). Each patient, except for one, had two sites treated, resulting in a total of 29 treated areas. All subjects had Fitzpatrick I–III skin phenotypes and brown or black hair.

Topical anesthetic cream was applied to the treatment sites, if required. The sites were then shaved. Treatment, through a cooling device, was then undertaken using a millisecond 1064nm Nd:YAG laser. Laser energy was delivered through a 2mm diameter spot size, with 30ms pulse duration and a fluence of 125–130J/cm$^2$ for facial hair or 150J/cm$^2$ for non-facial hair. Post-treatment care consisted only of ice packs, if desired.

Both physician and subject evaluated several parameters immediately following treatment and at follow-up visits. The degree of hair reduction (on a scale of 0–100%) was judged by physician and subject at 1 week, 1 month, and 3 months after treatment. Patients also rated their satisfaction on a five-point scale (1=worse; 5=excellent) at 1 week, 1 month, and 3 months. Adverse effects were monitored at each encounter. At 3 months, investigators determined whether treatment was considered a success on a basis of 30% reduction in hair density, no unanticipated adverse effects, no unresolved symptoms or adverse effects, and satisfaction rating by the subject of at least 3.

The physician assessment of hair reduction showed an overall 31% reduction at day 7, 52% reduction at day 30, and 59% reduction at day 90. The subject assessment of hair reduction was 23% at day 7, 45% at day 30, and 50% at day 90. The overall satisfaction rating of the subjects on a scale of 1–5 showed a mean score of 2.6 on day 7, 3.2 on day 30, and 3.3 on day 90. In all of these assessments, the perceived reduction of facial hair was greater than that of non-facial hair, although the differences were not found to be statistically significant. No complications or adverse effects were reported at any of the follow-up examinations.

## Kilmer (unpublished)

In a somewhat similar study, a millisecond Nd:YAG laser was evaluated using 15–30ms pulse durations and fluences of 50–60J/cm$^2$ (S Kilmer, personal communication). Twenty-five subjects with a total of 100 treatment sites were included. Skin phenotypes I–V were evaluated; anatomic sites included the face, arms, axillae, bikini area, and back. Response was assessed 3 months after a single treatment. The median hair count reduction 3 months after a single treatment was 32% for treatment parameters of 60J/cm$^2$ and 30ms; 24% for the treatment parameters of 50J/cm$^2$ and 15ms. The epidermal response 1 day after treatment included erythema, edema, and infrequent blistering. At the 3-month follow-up visit, minimal hyperpigmentation was noted in only 5 of the 100 treated sites. No hypopigmentation was noted.

## Aspects Not Yet Assessed

Whether multiple-session millisecond Nd:YAG laser treatment leads to better long-term results when compared with nanosecond Q-switched Nd:YAG laser treatment has yet to be determined.

# AVAILABLE Nd:YAG LASER SYSTEMS

## SoftLight (ThermoLase Corp., Carrollton, TX)

The SoftLight technique involves the combination of a topically applied exogenous chromophore carbon suspension used in conjunction with a 10ns, 1064nm, Q-switched Nd:YAG laser. Fluences of 1–3J/cm$^2$ are delivered through a 7mm spot size. The repetition rate of 10Hz leads to rapid laser treatments. This system is highly effective for temporary hair removal. The technology would not be expected to produce the permanent hair reduction seen with millisecond pulse duration lasers (Figure 7.3).

## MedLite IV (Continuum Biomedical, Dublin, CA)

This 8ns, 1064nm, Q-switched Nd:YAG laser is used without topically applied carbon suspension (Figure 7.4). Fluences of up to 8J/cm$^2$ are usually delivered

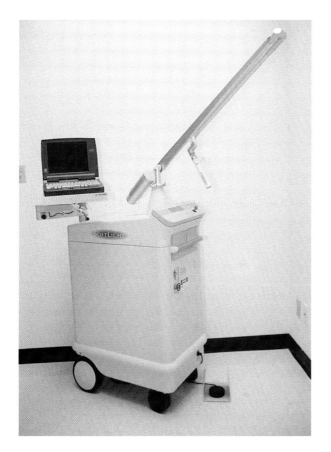

**Figure 7.3.** SoftLight laser used with topically applied carbon suspension

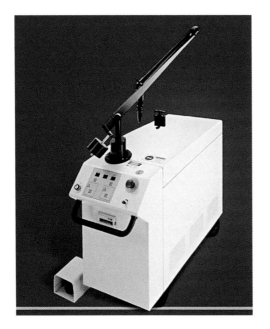

**Figure 7.4.** MedLite IV laser

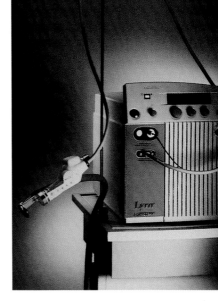

**Figure 7.5.** Lyra millisecond Nd:YAG laser

through a 4mm spot size. The repetition rate of 8Hz leads to rapid laser treatments. This system is highly effective for temporary hair removal. This technology would not be expected to produce the permanent hair reduction seen with millisecond pulse duration lasers.

## Lyra (Laserscope, San Jose, CA)

This is a millisecond Nd:YAG laser. Fluences up to $200J/cm^2$ with pulse durations varying between 10 and 100ms are delivered with a spot size up to 5mm (Figure 7.5). A scanner is provided and thermal damage is limited through contact cooling.

## CoolGlide (Altus Medical, Foster City, CA)

This laser is a 10–100ms Nd:YAG laser. Fluences up to $100J/cm^2$ are delivered through a $1 \times 1cm$ spot size. Contact precooling is provided (Figure 7.6).

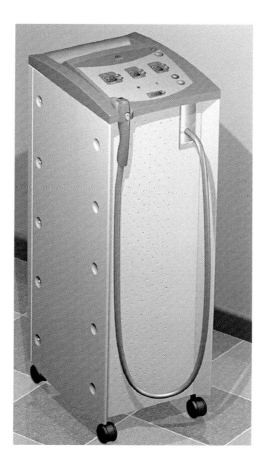

**Figure 7.6.** CoolGlide millisecond Nd:YAG laser

# MY APPROACH

I have found the nanosecond Q-switched Nd:YAG lasers to be highly effective in inducing temporary short-term hair removal. Although initially it was suggested that hair waxing aided in allowing the topical carbon suspension to penetrate deeper into hair follicles, there is no scientific proof that waxing makes any contribution to the final result. Skin cooling is not required when a nanosecond laser is used. This contrasts with the need for some form of epidermal cooling when virtually all millisecond lasers are used. The treatment technique using a nanosecond Q-switched Nd:YAG laser requires preoperative shaving of the treatment site. This reduces treatment-induced odor, prevents long pigmented hairs that lie on the skin surface from conducting thermal energy to the adjacent epidermis, and promotes transmission of laser energy down the hair follicle. When the technique is utilized with a topical carbon suspension, there is often a greenish hue to the area being treated when visualized through goggles. This is presumably due to the interaction between the 1064nm wavelength and the carbon chromophore. When the 1064nm Q-switched Nd:YAG laser is used without topical carbon chromophore, dark terminal hairs often turn white on laser impact. Usually no post-treatment crusting is noted. Erythema may vary from non-existant to significant in its extent. It is quite safe to treat individuals who have darker complexions with a nanosecond Q-switched Nd:YAG laser (Figures 7.7 to 7.27). It has been assumed that a millisecond ND: YAG laser system will produce better long-term results than a nanosecond system (Figures 7.7–7.33). Although our results, and those of Kilmer, would appear to be promising, long-term studies are required. Also, it would be expected that multiple treatments would lead to improved results. Although postinflammatory pigmentary changes from this laser are rare, such changes can be occasionally expected in some individuals with dark complexions.

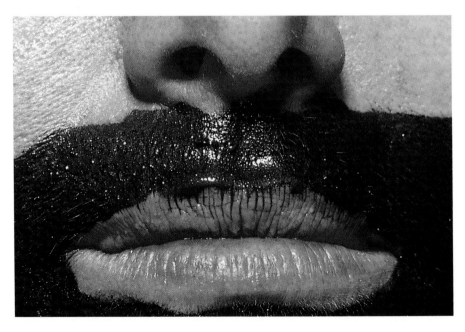

**Figure 7.7.** Carbon suspension applied to skin prior to laser irradiation with 1064nm Q-switched Nd:YAG laser

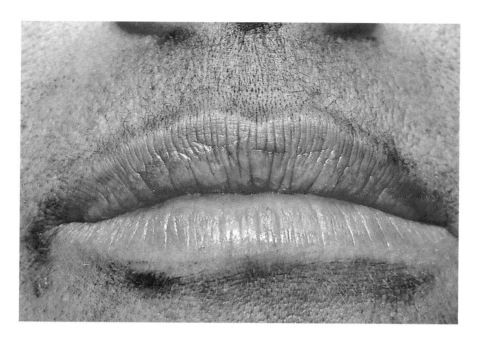

**Figure 7.8.** Immediately after laser irradiation of carbon suspension

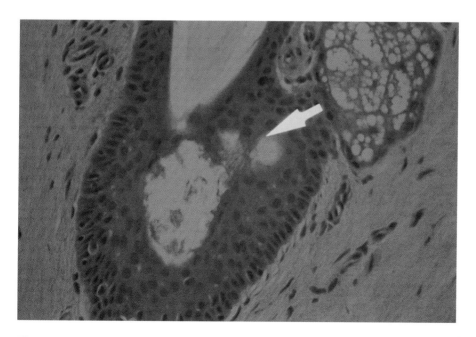

**Figure 7.9.** Vacuoles created within hair follicle after interaction of Q-switched Nd:YAG laser with topically applied carbon

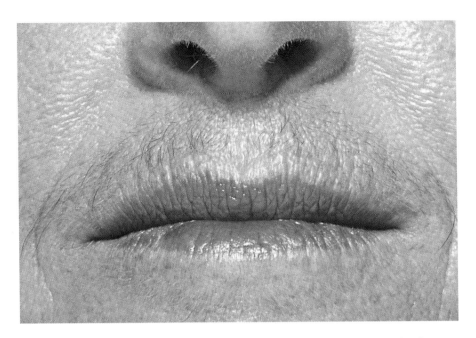

**Figure 7.10.** Hair on upper lip prior to treatment with topically applied carbon assisted Q-switched Nd:YAG laser

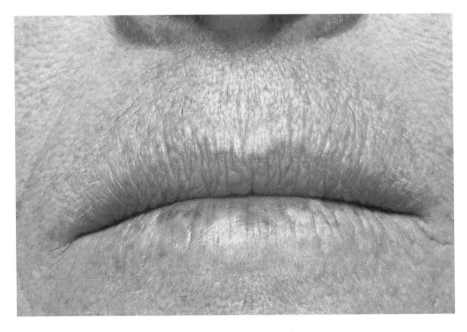

**Figure 7.11.** Minimal hair present on upper lip 2 months after treatment

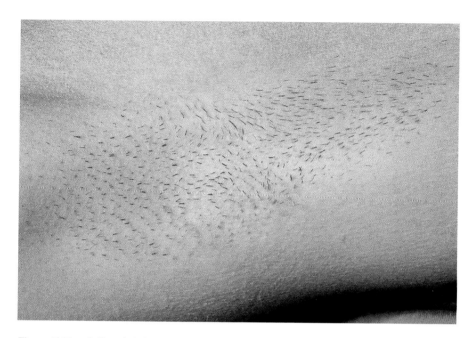

**Figure 7.12.** Axillary hair before treatment with topically applied carbon assisted Q-switched Nd:YAG laser

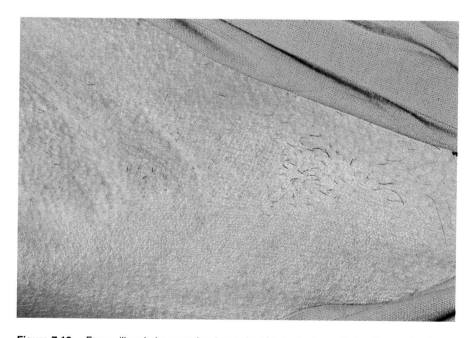

**Figure 7.13.** Few axillary hairs recurring 2 months after topically applied carbon assisted Q-switched Nd:YAG laser

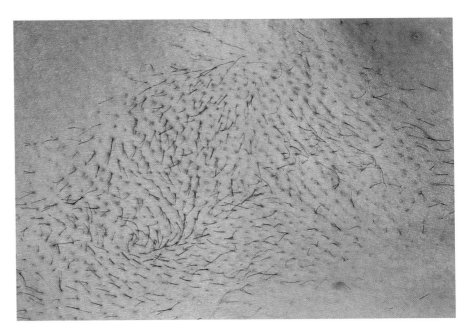

**Figure 7.14.** Axillary hair before treatment with topically applied carbon assisted Q-switched Nd:YAG laser

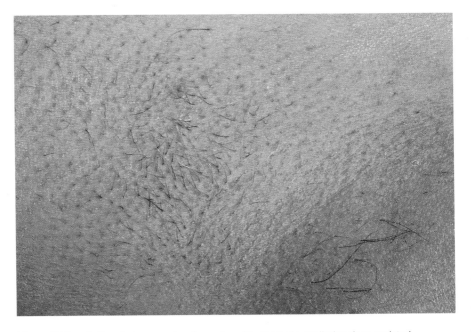

**Figure 7.15.** Axillary hairs recurring 3 months after topically applied carbon assisted Q-switched Nd:YAG laser

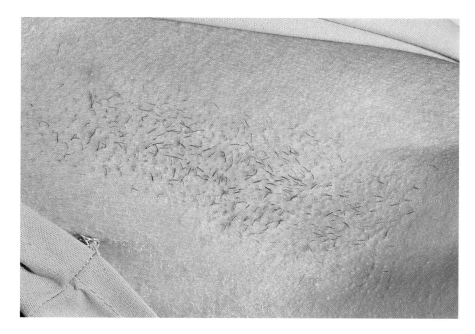

**Figure 7.16.** Axillary hair before treatment with topically applied carbon assisted Q-switched Nd:YAG laser

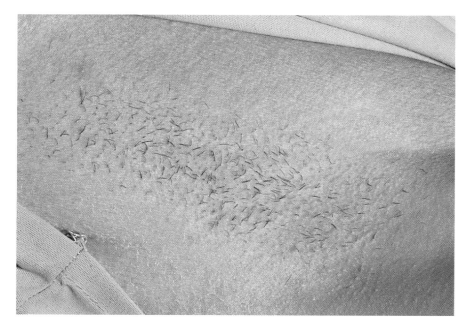

**Figure 7.17.** Axillary hairs totally recurred 3 months after topically applied carbon assisted Q-switched Nd:YAG laser

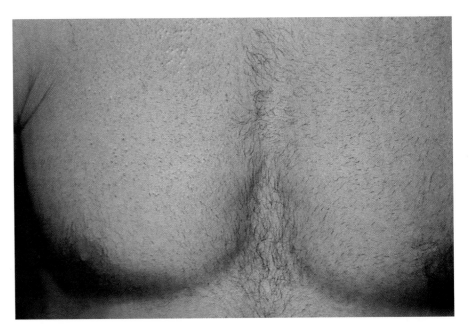

**Figure 7.18.** Chest hair before treatment with topically applied carbon assisted Q-switched Nd:YAG laser

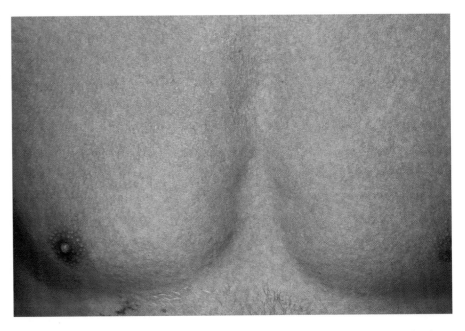

**Figure 7.19.** No chest hairs have recurred 1 month after topically applied carbon assisted Q-switched Nd:YAG laser

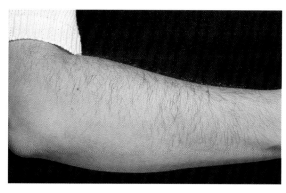

**Figure 7.20.** Arm hair before treatment with topically applied carbon assisted Q-switched Nd:YAG laser

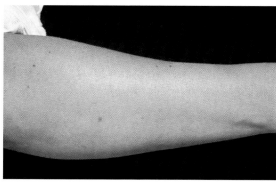

**Figure 7.21.** Immediately after treatment with topically applied carbon assisted Q-switched Nd:YAG laser

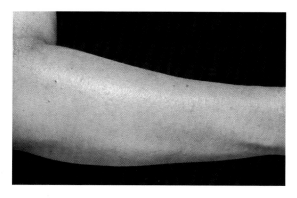

**Figure 7.22.** Arm hair 1 month after treatment with topically applied carbon assisted Q-switched Nd:YAG laser

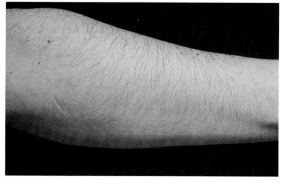

**Figure 7.23.** Arm hair 3 months after treatment with topically applied carbon assisted Q-switched Nd:YAG laser

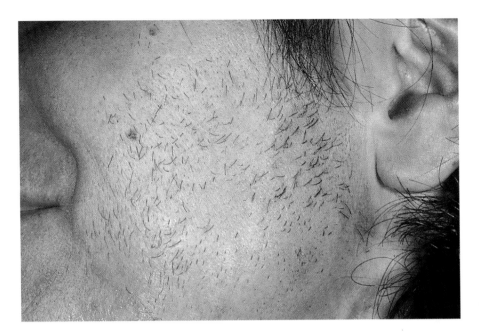

**Figure 7.24.** Left cheek before treatment with Q-switched Nd:YAG laser without carbon adjuvant

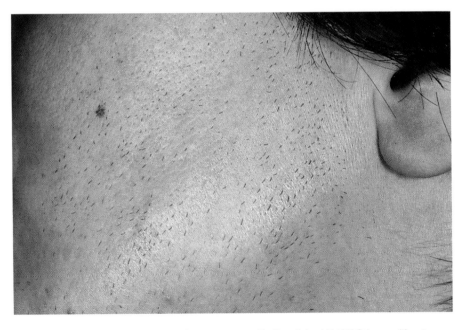

**Figure 7.25.** Left cheek 2 months after treatment with Q-switched Nd:YAG laser without carbon adjuvant

144

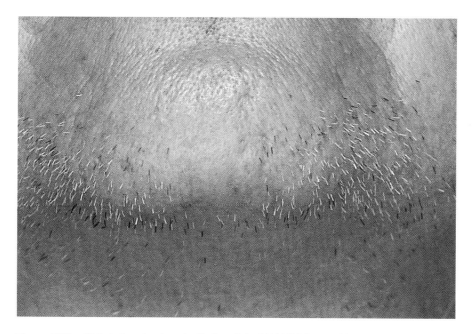

**Figure 7.26.** Chin before treatment with Q-switched Nd:YAG laser without carbon adjuvant

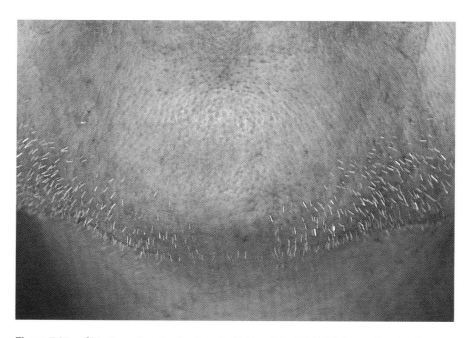

**Figure 7.27.** Chin 2 months after treatment with Q-switched Nd:YAG laser without carbon adjuvant. Note that only darker hairs have responded

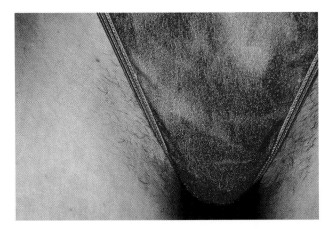

**Figure 7.28.** Bikini area before treatment with millisecond Nd:YAG laser hair removal

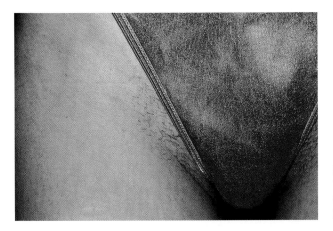

**Figure 7.29.** Bikini area 1 month after treatment with millisecond Nd:YAG laser hair removal

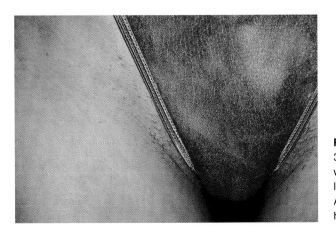

**Figure 7.30.** Bikini area 3 months after treatment with millisecond Nd:YAG laser hair removal. Approximately half of the hairs are gone

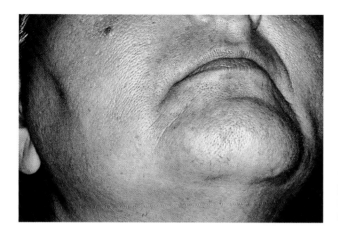

**Figure 7.31.** Chin hairs prior to treatment with millisecond Nd:YAG laser hair removal

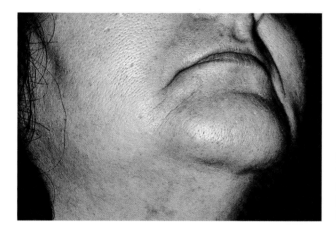

**Figure 7.32.** Chin 1 month after treatment with millisecond Nd:YAG laser hair removal

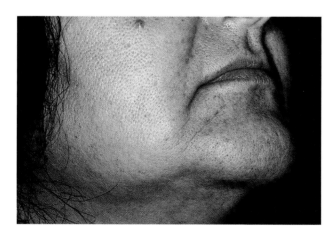

**Figure 7.33.** Chin 2 months after treatment with millisecond Nd:YAG laser hair removal. No perceptible hairs are present

# REFERENCES

1   Goldberg DJ, Littler C. Topical solution assisted laser hair removal. Lasers Surg Med 1995;15 (suppl 7):47.

2   Goldberg DJ, Littler CM, Wheeland RG. Topical suspension assisted Q-switched Nd:YAG laser hair removal. Dermatol Surg 1997;23:741–5.

3   Goldberg DJ. Topical suspension assisted laser hair removal: treatment of axillary and inguinal regions. Lasers Surg Med 1996;16 (suppl 8):34.

4   Nanni CA. Alster TS. A practical review of laser-assisted hair removal using the Q-switched Nd:YAG, long-pulsed ruby, and long-pulsed alexandrite lasers. Dermatol Surg 1998;24:1399–1405.

5   Bencini PL, Luci A, Galimberti M, et al. Long-term epilation with long-pulsed Neodymium:YAG laser. Dermatol Surg 1999;25:175–8.

6   Goldberg DJ. Evaluation of a long-pulse Q-switched Nd:YAG laser for hair removal. Dermatol Surg 2000;26:109–13.

# 8 INTENSE PULSED LIGHT

## KEY POINTS

(1) Intensed pulsed light is a non-laser light source
(2) The wavelengths delivered are between 590 and 1100nm
(3) Filters are used to choose delivered wavelengths
(4) There are myriad choices of pulse durations
(5) The risk profile is similar to visible light lasers
(6) There is greater diversity in choice of parameters than is seen with most lasers; correspondingly the learning curve is greater than that seen with lasers
(7) Millisecond high fluence systems have been cleared by the US FDA for permanent hair reduction

## BACKGROUND

Non-laser induced selective photothermolysis has become an accepted method of treating a wide gamut of vascular legions. This noncoherent, polychromatic light source can be 'tuned' to provide a variety of wavelengths, fluences, and pulse durations. Non-laser induced selective photothermolysis for hair removal has also been utilized with a filtered flashlamp, intense, pulsed light source (IPL) (Figure 8.1). Such a light source, when used for hair removal, delivers non-coherent light in the 590–1200nm range. The light is delivered in divided synchronized millisecond pulses separated by short thermal relaxation intervals for protection of epidermal melanin. The light is focused by a reflector and transmitted through a set of filters that determine its spectral characteristics. With non-laser light sources, a variety of parameters must be chosen. These include the spectrum of delivered wavelengths as determined by cut-off filters, number of delivered pulses, pulse duration in milliseconds, delay between pulses in milliseconds, and delivered fluence. The

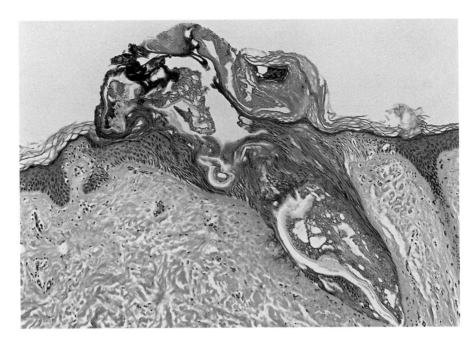

**Figure 8.1.** Histologic response immediately after IPL treatment. Significant thermal damage to the follicle is noted, with relative sparing of epidermis. No damage to surrounding dermis is noted

cut-off filters are utilized to tailor the spectrum of light to the skin type and hair color of the patient. The filter cuts off part of the emitted light, so that only wavelengths longer than the filter value pass to the treated hair and skin. As an example, a 615nm filter will only allow wavelengths greater than 615nm to be emitted. In general, the higher cut-off filters are utilized in individuals with darker complexions. The light is usually applied to the skin through a rectangular light guide. Cool gel and a bracketed cooling device have been used to cool the skin.

# CLINICAL STUDIES

The first published report of IPL use in hair removal documented successful long-term removal of terminal beard hairs in two transsexual patients.[1] Biopsies demonstrated atrophy of entire follicles, with no scarring at the skin surface. At 6 months, following a large number of treatments (13 and 41, respectively), no pigmented or textural skin changes were noted. Hair was found to be virtually absent.

Gold et al.[2] published the first significant series of patients treated with IPL. They evaluated hair removal efficacy in 31 subjects (3 men, 27 women, and 1 transsexual). Patients ranged in age from 14 to 74 years. The majority were between 30 and 50 years of age. A total of 37 treated sites were evaluated. All sites were treated one time and evaluated 2, 4, 8, and 12 weeks after treatment. Although a variety of anatomic sites were treated, the most common areas were the neck (27%), lip (22%), and chin (19%).

The treatment parameters were varied according to the pigmentation of the skin and treated hair. Four cut-off filters were used. They included 590, 615, 645, and 695nm. Delivered fluences ranged between 34 and 55J/cm$^2$. Energy was delivered in sequences of between two and five pulses, each pulse varying from 1.5 to 3.5ms in length. Interpulse delay time varied between 20 and 50ms. Generally, longer interpulse delays and multiple delivered pulses were used with higher fluences so as to better cool the skin between the pulses. In addition, larger numbers of pulses were used in darker skinned individuals for the same reason.

The study evaluated both immediate and later treatment responses. The immediate parameters were eliminated hair count, erythema, edema, purpura, burn, and post-treatment hair density. At follow-up visits, the authors analyzed the aforementioned parameters in addition to regrowth, change in hair color, scarring, textural changes, and pigmentary alteration.

Hair clearance was analyzed by placing responses into four quadrants: 0–25% clearance, 25–50% clearance; 50–75% clearance; and 75–100% clearance. Approximately one-third of the treated patients showed no clearance immediately after treatment. The remaining individuals were divided into the other three groups. Approximately one-fifth of the patients were in the top two quadrants.

At 2 weeks, there was a net shift of 10% of the population from the bottom quadrant to the top quadrant. This progression continued at the 4-week follow-up visit. At 4 weeks, only about 10% of the population was included in the lowest quadrant. The top two quadrants now represented about two-thirds of the population. The 8-week results were similar to those at 4 weeks. Approximately 60% of the patients were in the top two quadrants. Finally, at 12 weeks, the top two quadrants included 70% of the population.

The authors noted immediate post-treatment erythema in 70% of the patients. The only other immediate finding was edema, noted in 8% of the population. Two weeks after treatment, three cases of resolving blisters were reported. One case of hyperpigmentation was noted. No other complications were observed.

The authors followed patients for only 12 weeks. Thus, there could be no claim of long-term hair removal. In addition, patients were treated only one time. It would be expected that the results would be improved after multiple treatments. The authors did not delineate which Fitzpatrick phenotypes were treated: it might be expected that the complication rate would rise if darker skin types were treated.

Weiss et al.[3] expanded on the evaluation by Gold et al. of the IPL's hair removal efficacy. The former looked at not only the 3-month results after one treatment but also at hair removal efficacy 6 months after two treatments.

Twenty-eight sites on 23 subjects with Fitzpatrick skin types I–III were included in a study using a single IPL treatment. They were followed for 3 months. Another

56 sites on 48 subjects, with Fitzpatrick skin types I–V, were treated twice, with 1-month intervals between the two treatments. These individuals were followed for 6 months. Anatomic sites included in the double treatment protocol were facial regions (chin, submental region, neck, lip, ear, cheek, and preauricular locations) and non-facial regions (back, bikini area, thigh, shoulder, abdomen, and forearm). Treatment sites on the face averaged 25cm² in size, whereas treatment sites on the trunk averaged 50cm². Large areas could be treated due to the large spot size used (8 × 33mm or 10 × 45mm) delivered with each pulse.

The IPL treatment parameters utilized were a 2.8–3.2ms pulse duration for three pulses, with thermal relaxation intervals between pulses of 20–30ms. The 615 or 645nm cut-off filters were utilized, depending on skin type. Fitzpatrick type I and II subjects received treatment with the 615nm filter, types III and above with the 645nm filter. The triple pulses delivered a total fluence of 40–42J/cm². For the double treatment protocol, delivered fluences were increased only if the response to the first treatment was minimal. All other parameters remained unchanged.

The authors claimed to have used very conservative fluences for the single treatment protocol. At the first visit, immediate post-treatment mean hair clearance of 16% was recorded. This improved to 56% at weeks 2 and 4, and 54% at week 8, with a final 63% reduction at 12 weeks. These findings, suggestive of effective temporary hair removal, were consistent with those seen by Gold et al.[2] Of greater significance were the findings of the second study. In the double treatment protocol, immediate post-treatment clearance of 64% was achieved. These better results may be explained by the more aggressive parameters utilized in this second treatment protocol. At week 8, a 42% hair reduction was noted. At 6 months hair reduction was found to be 33%. In addition, many residual hairs were reduced in diameter. It is observations such as these which emphasize the importance of looking beyond simple hair counts in determining hair removal efficacy. Simple hair counts alone may be deceiving. Some patients in the study by Weiss et al. appeared to be excellent clinical responders even with hair counts reduced only by 33%. Because observed hairs were often much smaller in hair shaft diameter, they were less visible.

The expected post-treatment erythema, in the second study, was seen in 92% of patients. Urticarial edema around the hair follicles was noted immediately in 72% of treated individuals. Two sites developed a vesicle, which healed with no sequelae but led to several weeks of hypopigmentation. Approximately 12% of patients experienced some areas of crusting lasting several days to 1 week. Resultant hypo- and hyperpigmentation, lasting for 4–8 weeks, occurred as a result of the crusting. This cleared within 2 months in all cases. Of note is that patients who previously underwent electrolysis reported far less pain with IPL.

Examination of body study groups revealed maximal hair count reduction, at all sites, between 2 and 3 months after treatment. Partial regrowth of hair was observed at 6 months at all body sites. The authors suggested that this could be explained by the well-recognized, non-synchronous cyclical hair growth seen at different body locations. Another plausible explanation could also be invoked. It may be that the hair growth centers are merely damaged by IPL, or laser treatment, but not destroyed. It is also possible that some hairs simply do not respond to treatment.

Selim et al. have compared the results of IPL delivered in three different manners. (MM Selin, ME Flor, TA Johnson, BD Zelickson, personal communication). In one study, IPL treatment was delivered using a machine that had software that, although designed for spider vein treatments, could be utilized to treat unwanted hair. In a second study, a similar IPL device, with software designed specifically to treat unwanted hair, was utilized. In addition, the authors, in a third study, evaluated the effect of a particular bracketed cooling device during the treatments.

All subjects were Fitzpatrick skin phenotypes II–III. The first group consisted of 82 subjects, the second group 58, and the third group 20 subjects. Treatment areas included the face, neck, axillae, legs, bikini area, and back. All patients received one or more treatments. A variety of cut-off filters were utilized to optimize appropriate wavelength use. Fluences varying between 32 and 45J/cm² were used and delivered in double or triple pulses.

In the first study, 82 subjects (13 men, 60 women, 9 transsexual), ranging in age between 19 and 69 years (mean age of 35), were treated. From this group, 56 were seen in 1- to 5-month follow-up, while 13 were seen at between 6 and 16 months after treatment. The investigators noted better clearance in the 6 to 16-month group in Fitzpatrick skin type II (28% average clearance) compared with the Fitzpatrick skin type III group (16% average clearance). There was also an increase in clearance with subsequent treatments. In addition, hair removal was most efficient in darker hairs, compared with lighter hairs. The legs and bikini area showed the most clearance, the back the poorest results. One patient developed hyperpigmentation and one patient developed hypopigmentation. In both instances the pigmentary changes resolved within 6 months.

In the second study, 58 subjects (11 men, 41 women, 6 transsexual) were treated. The age range was 20–72 years (mean age of 38). Thirty-three subjects were seen in 1- to 5-month follow-up, while 17 subjects were seen at 6- to 16-month intervals. In this study, similar to the first study's findings, there was greater clearance in Fitzpatrick skin type II compared with Fitzpatrick skin type III. Type II subjects showed 64% clearance; skin type III showed 36% clearance. The reason for the disparity between the two sets of data was not provided. Nevertheless, greater improvement was again noted with an increasing number of treatments. In addition, increased hair loss was noted with darker hair colors. The bikini area was again the anatomic area showing the best response; the back showed poorer results. The neck and face also showed good results; the axillae showed poor results. The authors also noted a change in hair texture from coarse darker hair to thin lighter hair. No pigmentary alterations were noted.

When the investigators evaluated the effect of an IPL bracketed cooling device, in the third study, they noted a substantial reduction in treatment discomfort. However, the cooling device had no effect on the actual efficacy of treatment. There was also less blistering when the cooling device was utilized. Such a finding would be expected from any cooling device that protects the epidermis from thermal damage.

The above-mentioned studies were all performed with IPL devices developed by ESC Medical. In a study using a related IPL device not available in the USA, Bjerring[4] noted 46.8 hair removal reduction 6 months after three treatments given at 2-month intervals. These results, with the Ellipse IPL, compared with only a 6.3% reduction following similar treatments with a normal mode ruby laser. Troilus (A Troilus, personal communication), who noted an 87% IPL-induced clearance 4 months after four treatments, was able to show better results.

# AVAILABLE INTENSE PULSED LIGHT SYSTEMS

## EpiLight (ESC/Sharplan, Norwood, MA)

This intense pulsed light source is available worldwide (Figure 8.2). Utilized wavelengths vary between 590 and 1200nm. The light is delivered through a light guide. The most commonly used cut-off filters are 590, 615, 645, and 695.

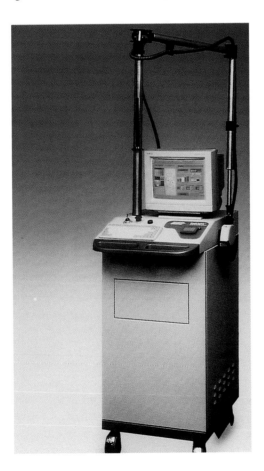

**Figure 8.2.** EpiLight IPL

Suggested fluences are 30–65J/cm² delivered in a double, triple, quadruple, or quintuple pulse sequence. Delivered pulse durations vary between 2.5 and 7.0ms with interpulse times between 1 and 300ms. Spot sizes up to 10 × 45mm can be delivered.

# Ellipse (Danish Dermatologic Development A/S, Hoersholm, Denmark)

This intense pulsed light source is marketed mostly in Europe and is not available in the USA (Figure 8.3). With this device, light is delivered through a 10 × 50mm spot size. Emitted wavelengths are somewhat different from the EpiLight, with a range of 600–950nm delivered at pulse durations of 1–50ms.

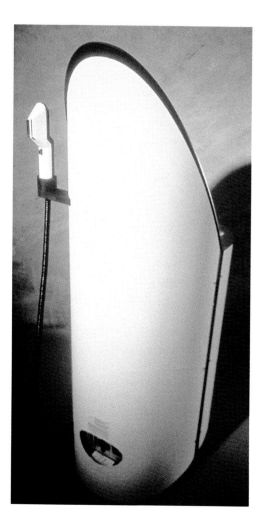

**Figure 8.3.** Ellipse IPL

## MY APPROACH

I have found intense pulsed light sources to be very useful in treating Fitzpatrick I and IV skin phenotypes. The IPL technique can also be used to improve hair-induced folliculitis (Figures 8.4 to 8.50). Although the EpiLight IPL source is FDA cleared in the USA for Fitzpatrick skin phenotype V (and similarly licensed in other countries), we have found that the incidence of postinflammatory changes may be too high for practical use in some of these individuals. Because red hair, with its associated pheomelanin, absorbs visible light best in the 400–600nm range, a 590nm filter is used in these patients so as to allow wavelengths of 590nm and above to be released. Fitzpatrick skin phenotypes II and III with dark terminal hair are best treated with the 615 or 645nm filters. Finally, Fitzpatrick IV individuals are treated with a 695nm filter. Such a filter skews emitted light towards the 800–900nm range for greater safety in these darker skinned individuals. In choosing emitted pulse durations, the anecdotal evidence points to shorter pulse durations being more helpful for finer hairs, while longer pulse durations appear to have greater efficacy in treating thicker hairs. In addition, longer pulse durations, because of their epidermal pigment sparing capacity, are chosen for darker skin phenotypes. The choice of the pulsing mode and interpulse times are also dictated by complexion. Darker complexions are usually treated with a double/triple pulse and longer interpulse times, in comparison with the parameters chosen with lighter skin complexions. As is true for all lasers used for hair removal, the higher the fluences, the better the results. The fluence chosen should be as high as can be tolerated without creating an epidermal blister.

The treatment technique commences with preoperative shaving of the treatment site. This reduces treatment-induced odor, prevents long pigmented hairs that lie on the skin surface from conducting thermal energy to the adjacent epidermis, and promotes transmission of laser energy down the hair follicle. My experience with the EpiLight light source has shown the greatest safety when both a coupling gel and the accompanying bracketed cooling device are utilized. Usually, postoperative perifollicular edema and erythema is noted. The treated hairs sometimes appear darker after treatment and usually fall out of the follicle 1–4 weeks after treatment. Retreatments are usually undertaken at 2- to 5-month intervals. In darkly pigmented or heavily tanned individuals, it may be beneficial to use topical hydroquinones and meticulous sunscreen protection for several weeks prior to the treatment in order to reduce inadvertent injury to epidermal pigment. Individuals with recent suntans should not be treated until pretreatment hydroquinones have been utilized for at least 1 month. Postinflammatory pigmentary changes still are to be expected in individuals who have darker complexions.

Intense pulsed light, when used with almost all fluences, can lead to temporary hair loss at all treated areas. However, choosing appropriate anatomical locations, utilizing higher fluences, and providing multiple treatments will increase the likelihood of permanent hair reduction. Even though permanent hair loss is not to be expected in all treated individuals, lessening of hair density and thickness are common findings.

The ideal treatment parameters must be individualized for each patient, based on clinical experience and professional judgment. The novice, when treating individuals

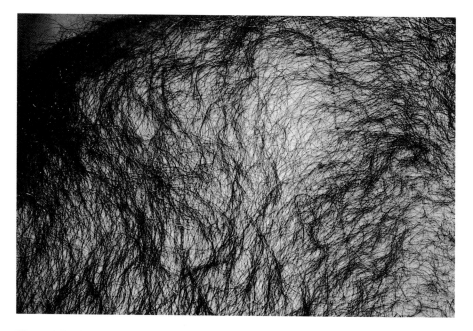

**Figure 8.4.**   Male back before treatment with IPL

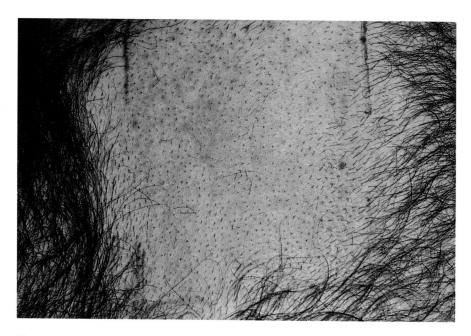

**Figure 8.5.**   Male back immediately after treatment with IPL. Note expected post-treatment erythema

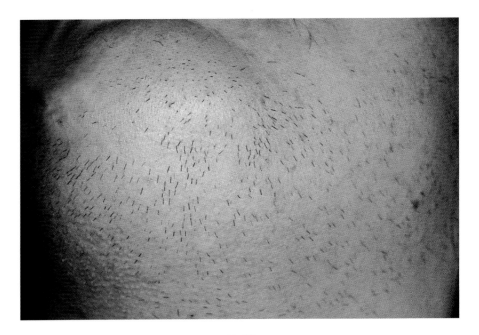

**Figure 8.6.** Hirsute chin before treatment with IPL

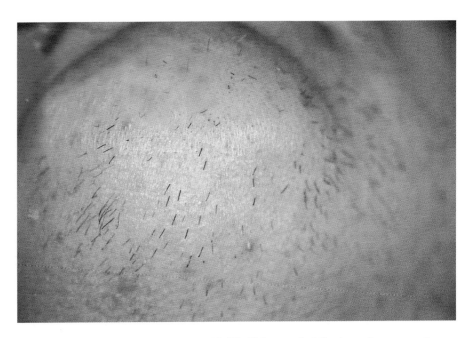

**Figure 8.7.** One month after treatment with IPL. Hairs usually fall out over the course of 1 month after treatment

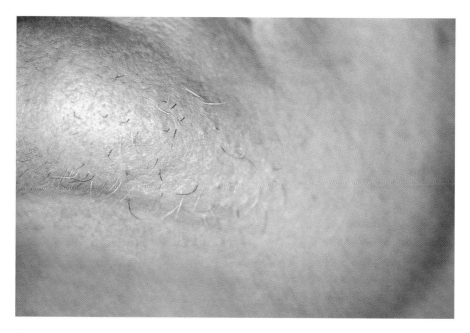

**Figure 8.8.** Postmenopausal woman before treatment with IPL. Note black and white hairs on chin

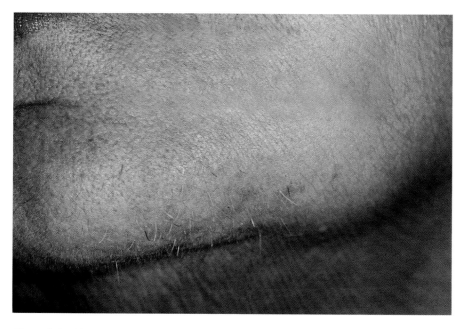

**Figure 8.9.** Postmenopausal woman 3 months after one treatment with IPL. Note most of the black hairs are gone. As would be expected, there is little response in non pigmented hairs

159

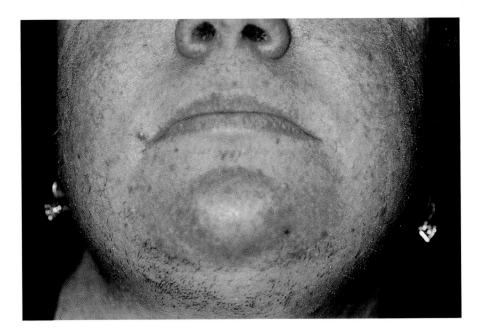

**Figure 8.10.** Dark terminal hairs on female chin

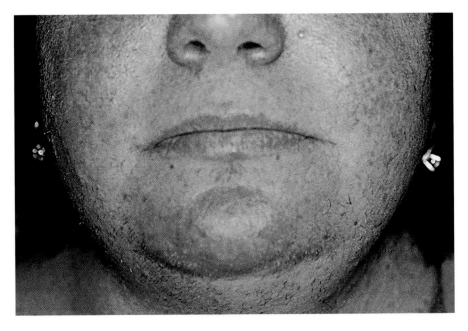

**Figure 8.11.** Excellent response 5 months after two treatments with IPL

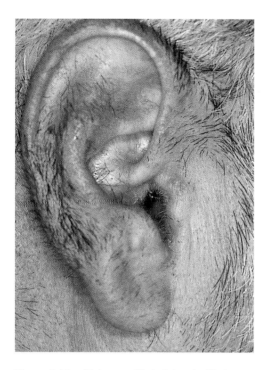

**Figure 8.12.** Male ear with dark terminal hairs

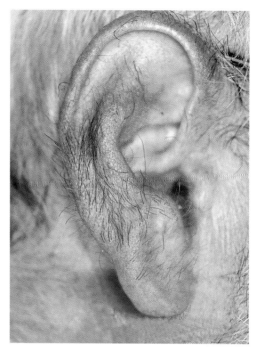

**Figure 8.13.** Some hair thinning noted 2 months after one treatment with IPL

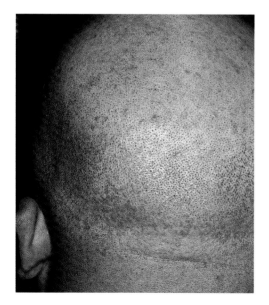

**Figure 8.14.** Type V male scalp hair before treatment with IPL

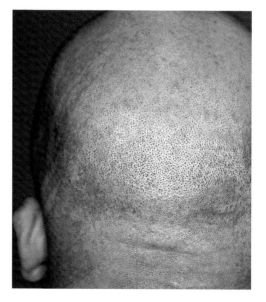

**Figure 8.15.** Mild thinning of hair noted 4 months after one session with IPL. As would be expected some postinflammatory hyperpigmentation is seen

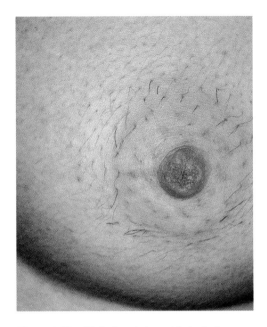

**Figure 8.16.** Right female breast hairs before treatment with IPL

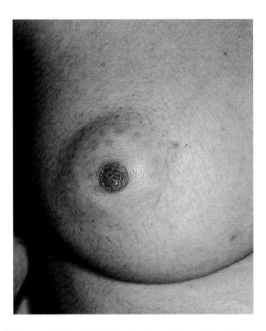

**Figure 8.17.** Right female breast 3 months after two sessions with IPL

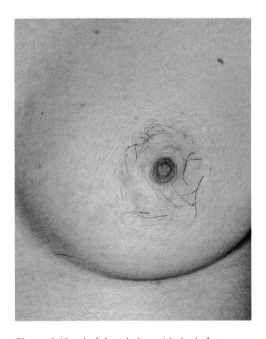

**Figure 8.18.** Left female breast hairs before treatment with IPL

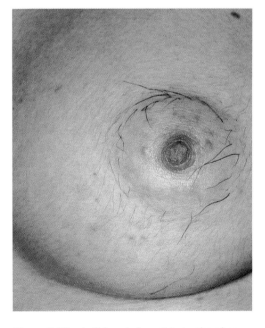

**Figure 8.19.** Left female breast 3 months after one session with IPL. Almost no improvement is seen. Multiple sessions are required

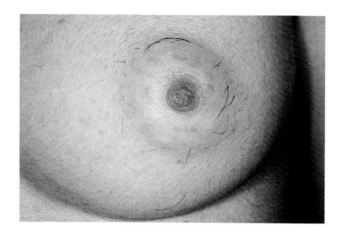

**Figure 8.20** Left female breast 3 months after two sessions with IPL. Almost no improvement is seen. Multiple sessions are required.

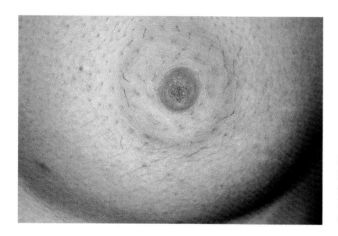

**Figure 8.21** Left female breast 3 months after three sessions with IPL. Improvement is now obvious.

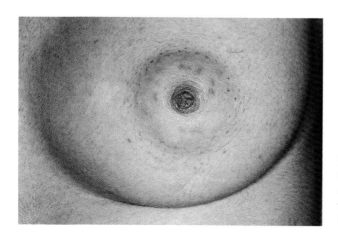

**Figure 8.22** Left female breast 6 months after five sessions with IPL. Only thin, lightly pigmented hairs persist.

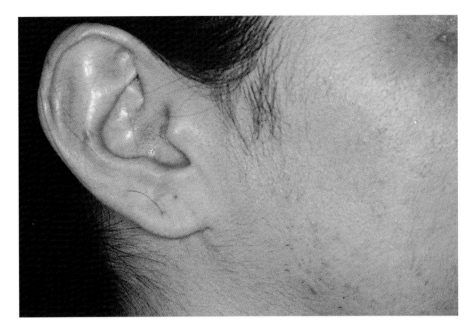

**Figure 8.23.** Right cheek hairs prior to treatment with IPL

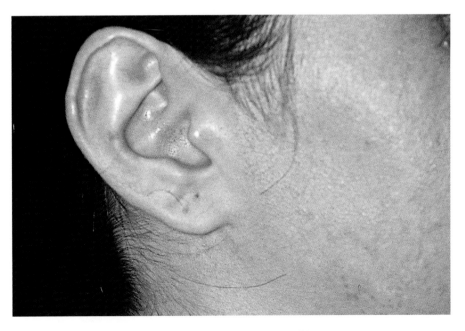

**Figure 8.24.** Right cheek 1 month after two treatments with IPL

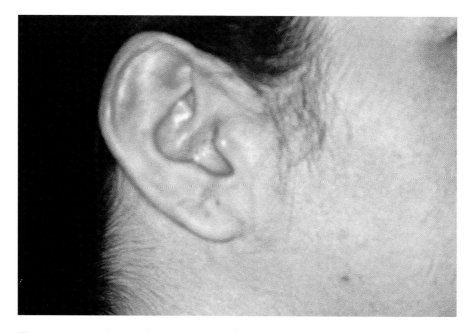

**Figure 8.25.**   Right cheek 3 months after two treatments with IPL

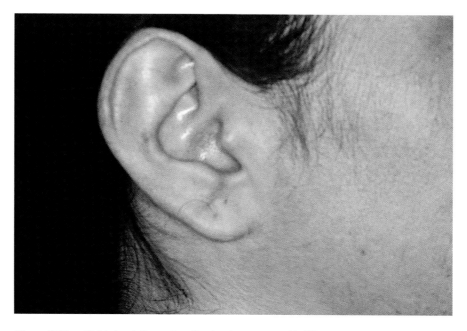

**Figure 8.26.**   Right cheek 6 months after two treatments with IPL

165

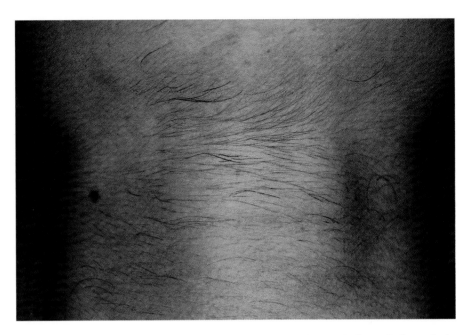

**Figure 8.27.** Neck before treatment with IPL. Note erythema from topically applied anesthetic cream

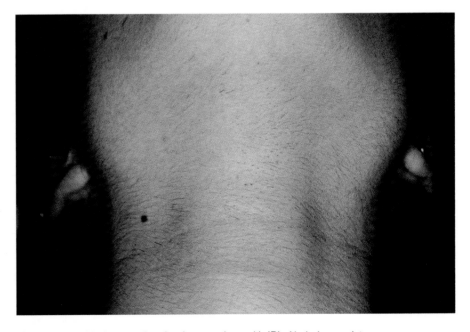

**Figure 8.28.** Neck 9 months after four sessions with IPL. No hairs persist

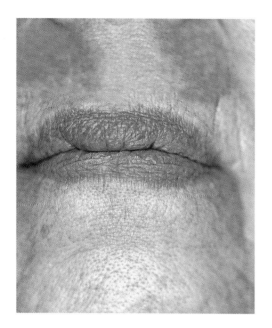

**Figure 8.29.** Several small hairs present immediately inferior to lip in this postmenopausal woman

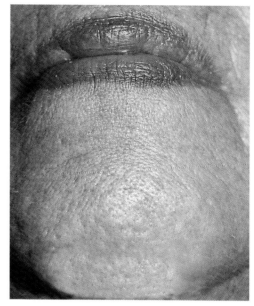

**Figure 8.30.** No hairs seen immediately inferior to lip in this postmenopausal woman 3 months after one treatment with IPL

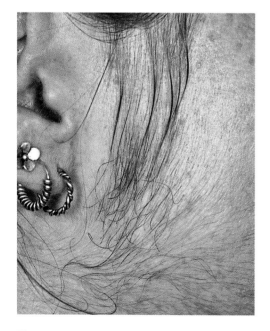

**Figure 8.31.** Red hairs present on right cheek

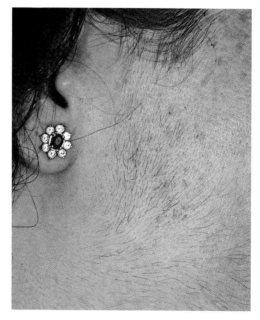

**Figure 8.32.** Marked thinning of hairs 6 months after three treatments with IPL using a 590nm cut-off filter

167

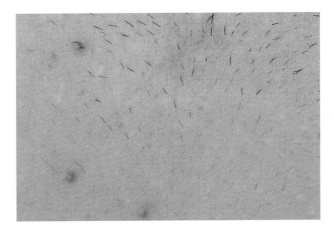

**Figure 8.33.** Hirsute female chest prior to treatment with IPL

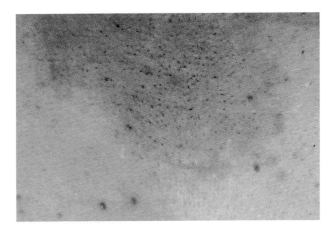

**Figure 8.34.** Erythema and perifollicular edema seen after treatment with IPL

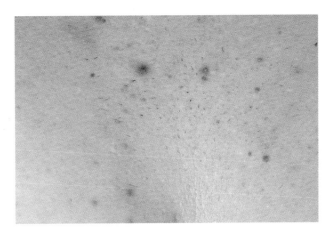

**Figure 8.35.** Minimal amount of hair present 2 months after treatment with IPL

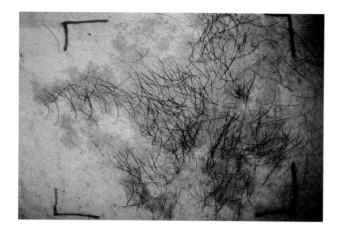

**Figure 8.36.** Hairs of Becker's nevus prior to treatment with IPL

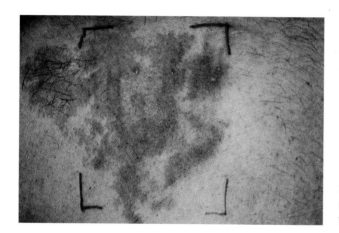

**Figure 8.37.** Erythema noted immediately after treatment with IPL

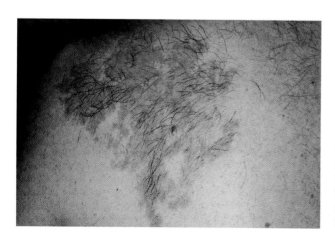

**Figure 8.38.** Six months after one treatment with IPL. All hairs appear to have regrown but are thinner than prior to treatment

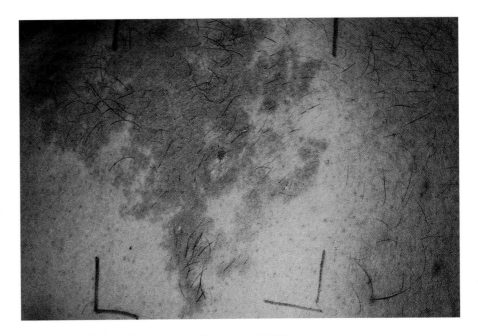

**Figure 8.39.** Six months after second treatment with IPL

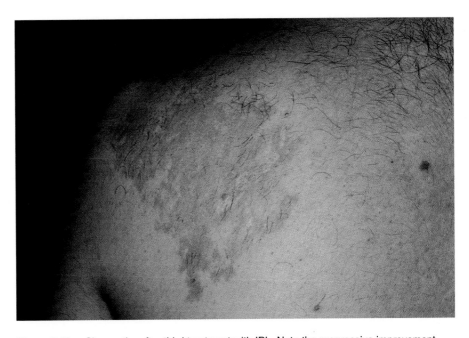

**Figure 8.40.** Six months after third treatment with IPL. Note the progressive improvement

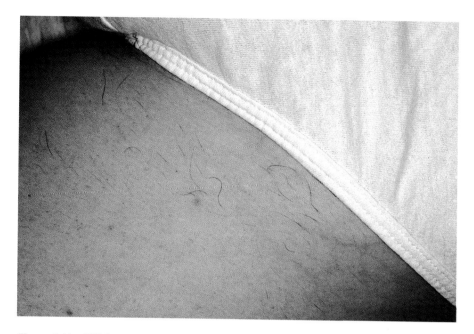

**Figure 8.41**   Bikini area prior to treatment with IPL.

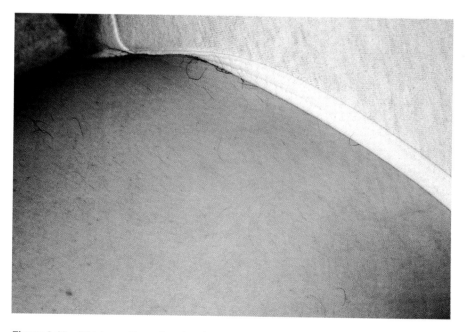

**Figure 8.42**   Bikini area 5 months after three treatments with IPL.

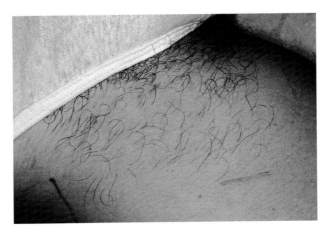

**Figure 8.43.** Bikini area prior to treatment with IPL

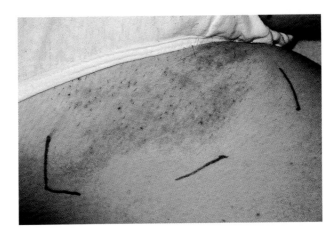

**Figure 8.44.** Perifollicular erythema and edema noted immediately after treatment with IPL

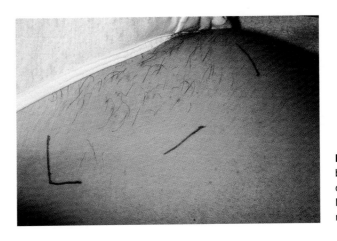

**Figure 8.45.** Hairs in bikini area 4 months after one treatment with IPL. Minimal improvement was noted

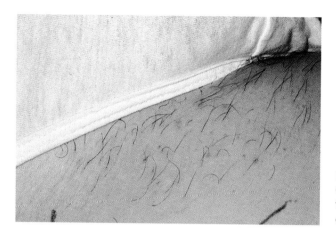

**Figure 8.46.** Bikini area 6 months after two treatments with IPL. Most of the hairs have regrown

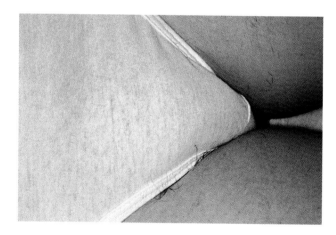

**Figure 8.47.** Bikini area 6 months after four treatments with IPL. Almost no hair is present

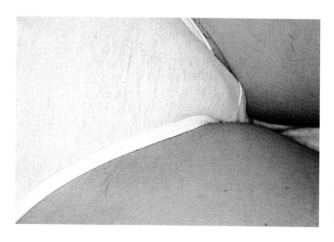

**Figure 8.48.** Bikini area 12 months after four treatments with IPL. Only a small number of fine hairs are noted

173

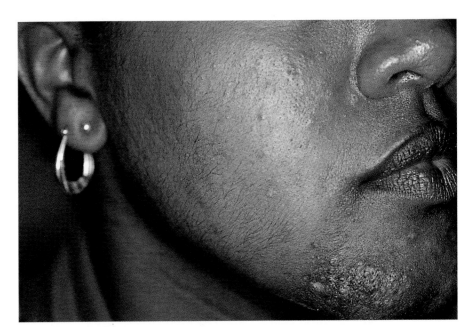

**Figure 8.49.** Significant folliculitis, postinflammatory hyper- and hypopigmentation in Fitzpatrick V skin phenotype prior to treatment with IPL

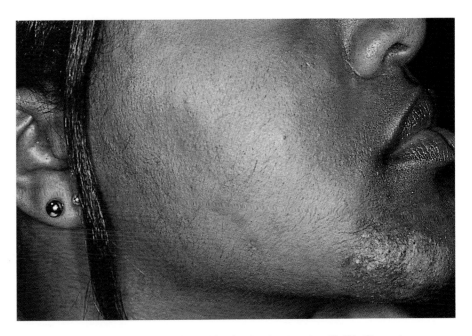

**Figure 8.50.** Mild improvement in folliculitis after two treatments with IPL. Pigmentary changes persist

who have darker complexions, may wish to undertake several individual test pulses at an inconspicuous site with a lesser fluence. The delivered energies may then be slowly increased. Undesirable epidermal changes such as whitening and blistering are to be avoided.

Prolonged and permanent hair loss may occur following the use of the intense pulsed light device. However, as with lasers, great variation in treatment results can be seen. No permanent skin change, depigmentation, or scarring has thus far been reported in the literature. However, there are now anecdotal accounts of cases of rare IPL-induced scarring and such a risk must be recognized.

# REFERENCES

1   Raulin C, Werner S, Hartschuh W, et al. Effective treatment of hypertrichosis with pulsed light: a report of two cases. Ann Plast Surg 1997;39:169–73.
2   Gold MH, Bell MW, Foster TD, et al. Long term epilation using the EpiLight broad band, intense pulsed light hair removal system. Dermatol Surg 1997;23:909–13.
3   Weiss RA, Weiss MA, Marwaha S, et al. Hair removal with a non-coherent filtered flashlamp intense pulsed light source. Lasers Med Surg 1999;24:128–32.
4   Bjerring P. Ellipse pulsed light hair removal. Presented at 2nd Annual European Society for Lasers in Aesthetic Surgery, Oxford, England, March 1999.

# 9 COMPLICATIONS

## KEY POINTS

(1) Permanent complications may include hyper/hypopigmentation and scarring
(2) Scarring is rare, but patients should be warned of the risks
(3) Tanned skin is at greater risk for pigmentary complications
(4) Temporary blistering may occur and indicates that the treatment parameters may have not been correctly selected
(5) Temporary urticaria occurs in 10% of patients
(6) Temporary perifollicular edema and erythema are common

## THE MAJOR REASONS FOR COMPLICATIONS

Complications following laser hair removal are rare, however they can occur. Our knowledge of laser physics and the impact of laser and light sources on the skin supplies an explanation for such complications. The ideal wavelengths for effective hair removal of pigmented hairs appear to be between 600 and 1100nm; these are the wavelengths best absorbed by melanin. Because the epidermis also has high concentrations of melanin, the epidermis is also sensitive to light irradiation. Thus 'selective' photothermolysis and its role in hair removal represents a balance between heat elevation in the treated hair and in the absorbing epidermis.[1]

Although the spectral range of 690–1100nm would appear to be the ideal choice for removing hair that is much darker than the skin, longer wavelengths may be more helpful in damaging deeper hairs that are not much darker than the skin. However, there is greater absorption of hair and epidermal melanin by the shorter visible light wavelengths. Therefore, although ruby, alexandrite and diode lasers are extraordinarily well absorbed by the melanin contained within hair (ruby > alexandrite > diode), there will always be absorption by epidermal melanin. This may result in epidermal blistering with resultant risk of hyper/hypopigmentation and scarring (Figures 9.1 and 9.2). With

177

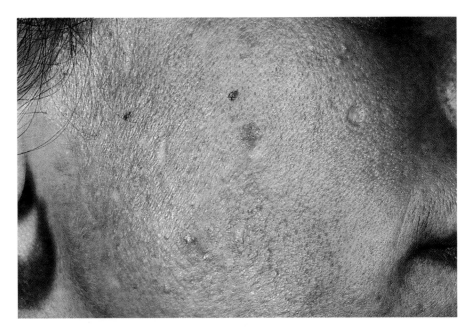

**Figure 9.1.** Facial hair in Fitzpatrick skin type IV prior to alexandrite laser with high fluences and no cooling of the skin

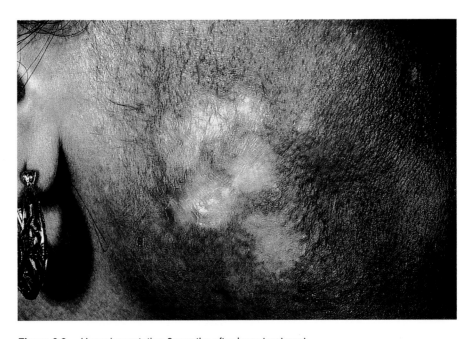

**Figure 9.2.** Hypopigmentation 6 months after laser treatment

sufficient epidermal cooling, however, one may be able to use these shorter wavelengths even when darker skin is treated. Cooling has been accomplished with cold gels, cryogen sprays and a variety of sapphire-tipped cooling devices.

When considering the appropriate timed pulse duration for the delivered energy, one must determine the diameter of treated hairs as well as the depth of penetration of the laser's emitted wavelength.[2] Thermal conduction during the laser pulse heats a region around the site of optical energy absorption. The spatial scale of thermal confinement and resultant thermal, thermomechanical, or thermoacoustic damage is strongly related to the pulse width of the emitted laser irradiation. Q-Switched, nanosecond, domain laser pulses effectively damage individual pigmented hairs within a hair follicle by confinement of heat solely at the level of the laser-impacted melanosomes. The thermal relaxation time of whole hair follicles is between 1 and 100ms. Thermal relaxation times of human terminal hairs of 130–250μm are thought to be between 10 and 50ms. In principle, a pulse duration that is shorter than the cooling time of hair, yet longer than the cooling time of the epidermis should be selected. This will enable the epidermis and small adjacent vessels to cool while the treated hair is being heated. For hair follicles larger than 130μm in diameter, the hair cooling time is longer than the epidermal cooling time (about 3–7ms). Therefore, choosing longer emitted pulses can enhance selectivity. Longer pulse widths, at least in theory, would allow more thermal conduction and damage to non-pigmented regions of the hair follicle, but would confine the thermal damage

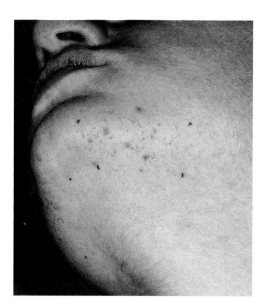

**Figure 9.3.** Left chin facial hair prior to laser treatment

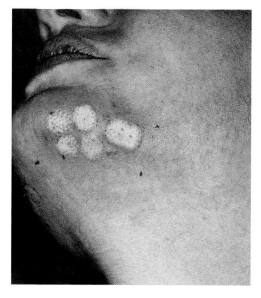

**Figure 9.4.** Chosen fluences were too high leading to immediate post-treatment epidermal whitening

179

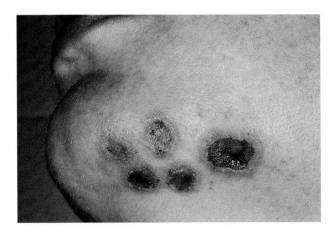

**Figure 9.5.** Left chin, 1 week after laser treatment. Epidermal blistering led to significant crusting

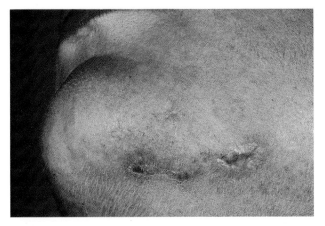

**Figure 9.6.** Left chin, 4 weeks after laser treatment. Scars are present

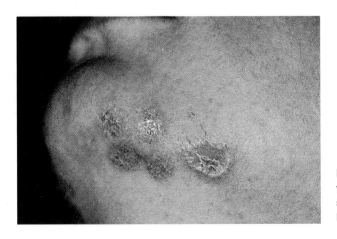

**Figure 9.7.** Left chin, with atropic erythematous scars 6 months after laser treatment

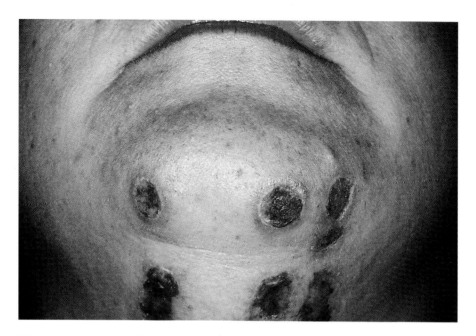

**Figure 9.8.** One week after treatment in a research protocol, where fluences were excessive and no epidermal cooling was provided

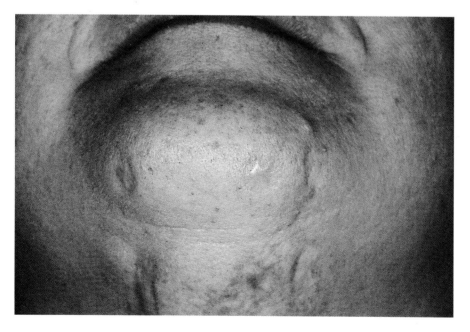

**Figure 9.9.** Six months after laser treatment. Scars are obvious

solely to the hair.[2] Thus, longer pulse durations lasers, all else being the same, may be safer in individuals with darker complexions. A shorter pulse may lead to greater epidermal heat and blistering, with resultant risk of hyper/hypopigmentation and scarring in these darker individuals.

The fluences used may also impact on efficacy. Higher delivered energies allow more photons to be delivered to the deeper regions of a hair follicle. Thus, with comparable wavelength laser systems, higher fluences usually lead to better results. Conversely, if delivered fluences are too high, significant thermal damage may ensue, with a resultant increase in thermal damage (Figures 9.3 to 9.9).

# SUN-TANNING

Even when safe parameters are chosen, recently tanned skin appears to be more photosensitive to laser light. If a tanned individual is treated with any of the visible light lasers or light sources (and perhaps even the near-infrared systems), increased melanin absorption occurs, leading to a greater risk of pigmentary changes and scarring (Figures 9.10 to 9.16). In addition, post-treatment sun-tanning can also lead to a greater risk of postinflammatory pigmentary changes[3] (Figure 9.17).

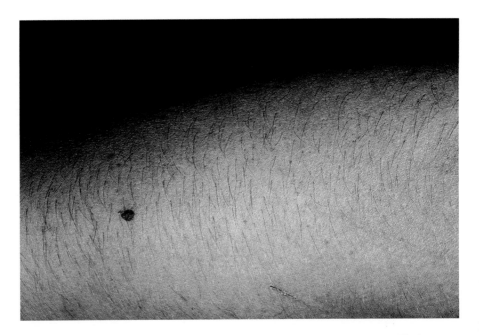

**Figure 9.10.** Recently sun-tanned arm in patient with Fitzpatrick skin phenotype III prior to treatment with laser

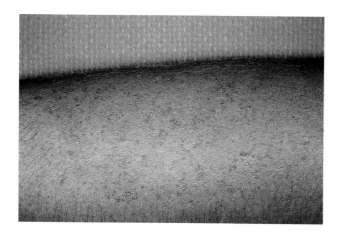

**Figure 9.11.** Immediate post-treatment. Minimal erythema is seen

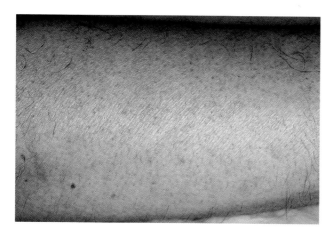

**Figure 9.12.** One day after laser treatment. Erythema appears to be resolved

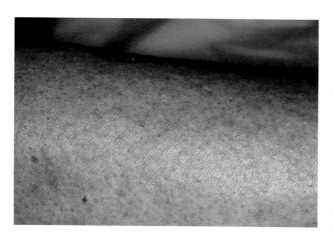

**Figure 9.13.** Mild blistering noted at day 2

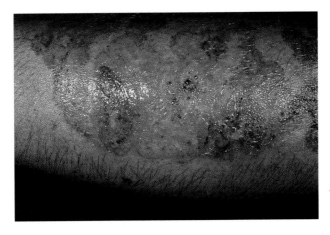

**Figure 9.14.** Epidermal denudation at day 3 in a patient with recent sun-tan

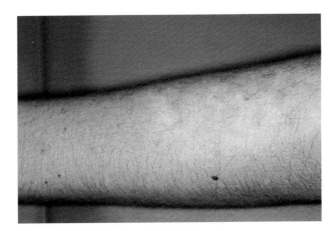

**Figure 9.15.** Hypopigmentation at 6 months after laser treatment

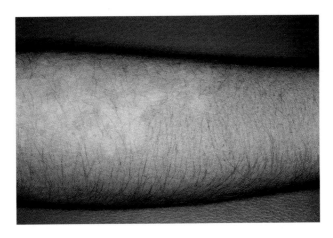

**Figure 9.16.** Hypopigmentation 12 months after laser treatment

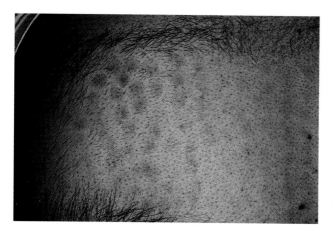

**Figure 9.17.** Postinflammatory hyperpigmentation of shoulder in male patient who sunbathed 2 weeks after laser treatment

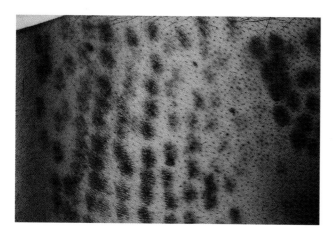

**Figure 9.18.** Exuberant laser response in densely haired male shoulder

# HIGH HAIR DENSITY

Anatomic areas that have increased hair density absorb laser light to a greater degree than do relatively less dense regions of hair. In such cases, it is better to use a lower fluence to lessen post-laser inflammation (Figure 9.18).

# URTICARIA

Approximately 10% of treated individuals have what appears to be a post-treatment urticaria-like response (Figures 9.19 and 9.20). It is not clear that such individuals have an atopic diathesis. Such individuals may be pretreated with oral antihistamines.

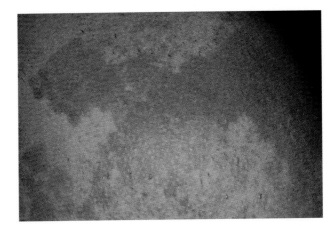

**Figure 9.19.** Immediate post-treatment urticarial response

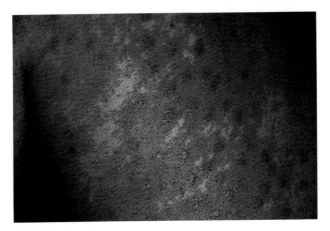

**Figure 9.20.** Immediate post-treatment urticarial response

# PERIFOLLICULAR EDEMA AND ERYTHEMA

It should be noted that perifollicular edema and erythema are common findings after laser hair removal (Figures 9.21 to 9.23). Such an endpoint is a desired effect with the millisecond laser/light source systems. This endpoint is often obscured in those patients with the aforementioned urticarial-like response.

# SCARRING

Scarring is always a possibility following any cosmetic procedure. It can happen without identifiable cause (Figures 9.24 and 9.25). This risk should be explained to the patient prior to the treatment.

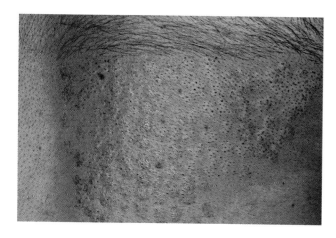

**Figure 9.21.** Immediate post-treatment perifollicular edema and erythema

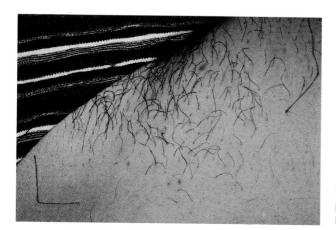

**Figure 9.22.** Bikini hair prior to treatment with intense pulsed light

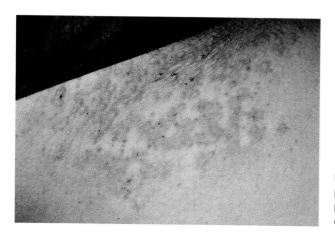

**Figure 9.23.** Immediate post-treatment perifollicular edema and erythema

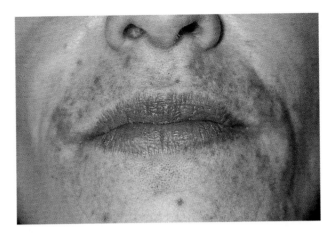

**Figure 9.24.** Typical post-laser perifollicular erythema and edema of upper lip

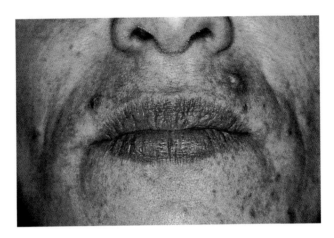

**Figure 9.25.** Hypertropic scars 6 months after laser treatment. No obvious cause was identified

# REFERENCES

1  Mainster SA, Sliney DH, Belcher D, et al. Laser photodisruptors. Damage mechanism, instrument design and safety. Ophthalmology 1983;99:973–91.
2  Dierickx CC, Grossman MC, Farinelli WA, et al. Permanent hair removal by normal mode ruby laser. Arch Dermatol 1998;134:837–42.
3  Hasan AT, Eagelstein W, Pardo RJ. Solar-induced postinflammatory hyperpigmentation after laser hair removal. Dermatol Surg 1999;25:113–15.

# 10 MARKETING A LASER HAIR REMOVAL PRACTICE

## KEY POINTS

(1) Laser services are now part of the mainstream of a cosmetic surgery practice and are increasingly being offered in other specialties' practices
(2) Marketing starts with high-quality therapy in a patient-friendly environment: presentation of services is important
(3) Promotion varies enormously in cost, depending on method, and should be rigorously assessed in terms of its success in attracting patients

## INTRODUCTION

As one reflects on the marketing of a laser hair removal practice, two striking observations become self-evident. First, laser services are no longer ancillary in any cosmetic practice. The revenue streams from a full service cosmetic surgery practice and an esthetic laser hair removal clinic can be equal. Because in many centers laser hair removal is delegated, it has been a tremendous addition to many practices. It expands the revenue base without the physician having to perform the services him or herself. Any time that one can develop such 'multipliers' in a business, there is a powerful opportunity to maximize revenue or free oneself to do other things. Secondly, the attendance at laser hair removal seminars and courses has shifted to include, in addition to the traditional esthetic medical specialists, internists, family physicians, obstetricians, gynecologists, practitioners of complimentary medicine, neurologists, and non-medical practitioners such as dentists, oral surgeons, chiropractors, estheticians, homeopaths and nurses.

Why have both the demographics of the attendees shifted and the popularity of laser hair seminars increased? Simply because of population shift and economic reality. At the same time that an increasingly affluent population enters into its prime spending years, all of medicine and allied health services have witnessed a major contraction in traditional insurance and health care reimbursements. The explosion in cosmetic surgery, laser skin care, and esthetic services has created an attractive market and source of additional revenue for all medical, allied health, and non-medical practitioners.

The marketing principles outlined in this chapter are general enough to be of benefit to any practitioner who wants to augment a laser hair removal practice. They are also specific enough that any practitioner who has purchased a laser or intense pulsed light hair removal system can benefit immediately from the chapter's advice. However, the principles are based on current permissible approaches to marketing esthetic procedures in the USA and should be read in the context of any existing legislation or professional restrictions in the reader's own country.

# WHAT IS MARKETING?

Most physicians starting a laser hair removal practice equate marketing with advertising. Most doctors are very good at spending money on advertising to make the phone ring but are very poor at marketing. Anyone can spend money to make the phone ring. That's not marketing, that's the easy part. Marketing is a summation of all the activities and procedures that a physician, as the provider of a product (your esthetic services), must perform/implement to deliver the product into the hands of the consumer. Advertising may only represent a very small or non-existent component of a practice's marketing plan. There are many yardsticks by which to measure a successful marketing plan, but profitability and return on investment (ROI) are the most important for practitioners of esthetic laser services. Concepts of medical marketing can be condensed into the '10 Ps' of medical marketing.

| The 10 Ps of Esthetic Medical Marketing | |
|---|---|
| 1. Physician | 6. Price |
| 2. Product | 7. Precision |
| 3. Plan | 8. Predictability |
| 4. People | 9. Profitability |
| 5. Place | 10. Pleasure |

# PHYSICIAN

In medicine, unlike some businesses, promotion can not be substituted for quality. The most important aspect of a profitable practice, and marketing that practice, is a quality physician. As doctors, our product is not a disposable plastic toy, where quality can be variable; ours must only be measured in excellent patient outcomes. We have an ethical and moral obligation to our patients, as physicians, to deliver quality esthetic health care and above all else 'do no harm'. Most businesses and their products are not bound by such intimate and ethical standards. We, as physicians delivering an esthetic service, can never compromise the well-being of our clients with our products.

Part of our role, as physicians delivering a laser hair removal service, is to know the product well. We must learn the basics of laser medicine, laser safety, wound healing, and hair biology. We must also keep up-to-date on the latest developments by going to meetings, reading journals, and maintaining our continuing medical education. We never must lose sight of our role as a physician. If we do, then all the other Ps of practitioner marketing are worthless.

# PRODUCT

Once one becomes a high-quality laser physician, the next step is the delivery of a quality hair removal product to the laser hair removal client. Deciding upon the right technology can be a very difficult decision. There are many difficult questions such as optimum fluence, pulse duration, wavelength(s), and skin cooling. It is inevitable that there will continue to be technology advances in optimizing the removal of unwanted hair. Features of laser or intensed pulse light systems that are important include:

(1) **Speed:** the faster the system (Hertz and spot size dependent) the more effectively you can work and the more affordable your service will be for your clients. The ability to offer laser hair removal quickly and affordably for large zones (backs and legs) has been a tremendous advance. It has opened a whole new area of demand that has been relatively unavailable to electrolysis.

(2) **Accuracy:** there is no point being very fast with a system if you, or your assistant, miss large areas which then require retreatment (as these additional sessions will have to be offered to the client free). Systems that employ computer-generated scanners or large delivered spot sizes offer tremendous accuracy. Both will minimize your 'missed zone' retreatment rate.

(3) **Service:** you will want to choose a laser company that will still be doing business in a year, provide quality service in a field, and whose technology has an excellent track record. Realistically, all systems will have some down time for repair and maintenance.

# PLAN

An excellent physician with a good laser hair removal system needs a plan. If one 'fails to plan – then one plans to fail'. Short of an actual business plan, there are three simple questions one must answer as part of a plan to implement laser hair removal into a practice.

## Market Analysis

If you are an obstetrician, dermatologist, or primary care physician with 10,000–20,000 patients in your roster, then you are in an ideal position to implement laser hair removal. Your initial market is your own patient roster. For other physicians, the practice base may not be large enough for it to be worthwhile, or there are only one-time patients. One may need to consider actively recruiting patients, through promotion, into the hair removal practice. There may be a need to conduct a quick (and easy) marketing analysis to determine the viability of your enterprise. The target market is women between 20 and 65 years old, making over $30,000 per year (for simplicity, all monetary units in this chapter are expressed in US dollars). To find out how many demographic matches live in your locale, simply call up any medium that you might be interested in advertising with (radio, newspapers, or magazines) and they will gladly send the market breakdown for your area (as they have already obtained this marketing analysis themselves). The following is an example of the simple analysis you will require.

(1) **City population:** 2 million.
(2) **Demographic matches** (target market): Women, 20–65 years, making over $30,000, say for example 680,000.
(3) **'2.5% Rule':** this is an advertising assumption, which states that, of a susceptible target market for a product, only 1/40 (2.5%) might respond to advertising for this product.
(4) **680,000 ÷ 40** = 17,000 potential clients; however, there will be other clinics, possibly 30, performing laser hair removal in your locale.
(5) **17,000 ÷ 30** = 567 clients = market share: the number of potential clients in your region that can be obtained from your advertisements. This does not include potential patients that may come from other hair removal clinics.

If the potential market share is 300 people or greater, then the region is not saturated. A profitable hair removal practice should result.

## Financial Modeling

If there are 500 clients in the clinic's market share, the average amount spent by clients is approximately $500 per visit. The average patient returns four times: 500 clients × $500 × 4 treatments = $1,000,000. Thus, if the laser hair removal clinic is converting maximally all potential patients into treatments, retreatments and word of mouth referrals, then a $1 million dollar/year laser hair removal practice should result. However, because physicians never convert anywhere near maximally (100%), most physicians will earn $50,000–100,000 after expenses.

## Marketing Plan

All the Ps in this chapter must be implemented for a successful marketing plan. A good marketing plan will keep the laser hair clinic profitable.

# PEOPLE

The first step is to become a well-trained, knowledgeable laser practitioner. Then one needs a quality, fast, accurate hair removal device. This is followed by a planning and marketing analysis that indicates there is a viable opportunity to generate additional revenue in one's local hair removal market. Only then is it time to consider the people who will be delivering the product. The people a physician hires to represent the esthetic laser service are the next most important critical resource, after the doctor and the product, in delivery of cosmetic laser hair removal. Remember, these are the people who will present, represent, and promote your hair removal product on the phone, in your office, and in the community.

This highly sales oriented position requires an outgoing, friendly, and persuasive individual. How does one hire these motivated outgoing types? They are in high demand. Obviously careful interviewing, references, and experience are necessary. Some practitioners have even hired human resource consultants to uncover the required sales traits and skills. In the final analysis, after the usual due diligence, interviewing, and reference checks, one often hires such individuals on gut instinct. A certain amount of luck is always required!

After hiring staff, the members of the staff must be empowered by teaching them about laser hair removal. This will allow them to sell the procedure. Give them phone scripts for new callers. Offer staff complimentary treatments. They will become the most enthusiastic supporters of the services. They will sell the hair removal product with a tremendous sense of conviction that the clients will sense.

Finally, remuneration is critical. Giving staff a feeling that they are sharing in the success always helps. Front desk staff (client service representatives), office managers, and laser technicians should always be paid a healthy base salary, commensurate with expertise and/or experience. One could advocate leaving room for bonus incentives based upon staff's ability to convert contacts to treatments. For the receptionist, it will be the number of calls (leads) for consultation; for the laser nurse it will be converting treatments to retreatments, and for the office manager, who oversees the whole process, it will be a bonus on the percentage of incremental increase in sales. These monthly bonuses must always be an acceptable percentage of the increasing bottom line. Some form of bonus remuneration will lead to a well-trained, happy, motivated staff.

# PLACE

The laser hair removal clinic will need a place for staff and technology. The clinic should always reflect the image of the provider (the physician), and the product. Remember people are paying for a service they cannot claim on insurance and they will expect a quality outcome that is also delivered in pleasant surroundings. There is competition for their 'hair removal dollars'. That does not mean you must have museum quality paintings hanging on the walls. However, it is important to pay careful attention to the 'look' and 'feel' of the clinic setting so as to maximize the positive impact upon your potential hair removal patients and make them feel at ease.

After providing for a careful, tasteful, image appropriate and coordinated approach to interior decorating, one must carefully plan all contact points with hair removal patients and create a positive image.

## The Waiting Room

Keep this a relatively small private area, with no more than one or two patients waiting at a time. Patients hate to feel 'herded' and do not like to wait; their time is as valuable as that of anyone else. Schedule clients so they have five minutes to settle into the atmosphere of the clinic. During this 'absorption phase', they should be informed (through brochures, videos, posters, prompts, guides, and product displays) of some of the other beneficial aspects of the cosmetic services offered.

As the clients arrive, greet them by name. They like to feel that you know them. Don't be afraid to offer a refreshment or snack (examples would include mineral or spring water, tea, coffee, or a light snack).

## The Consultation

The consultation or treatment, whether offered by a nurse or physician, should be part encouragement ('sales') and part informed consent. The positive side of laser hair removal should always be emphasized first. Once clients know about the procedure, benefits, and cost, the informed consent should include alternative treatments, advantages, disadvantages, and risks. The patient should have an opportunity to fully read the consent form, have any questions answered to their satisfaction, and should then sign each page of the consent document (indicating that it was read and understood).

A well-executed consultation and consent for hair removal should leave the client excited and hopeful about the potential results, well informed, understanding of the risks, and enthusiastic about going on to treatment.

## The Treatment Room

A 3 × 4 m room is ideal. Provide room for changing and reapplication of makeup. Never miss an opportunity to inform people of other cosmetic services during treatments. Posters, videos and motivated laser nurses can assist laser hair removal patients assess other available esthetic services.

# PRICE

The fees charged for laser hair removal services will vary according to the anatomic zone, type of practice, who delivers the service, laser speed, laser type, and competitive prices (the 'price-point') in the local laser hair removal market.

This last factor, price-point in the market, will likely be the most important influence in setting fees. In most markets there will be a fairly narrow range of prices charged for laser hair removal performed on lips, chins, armpits, legs, backs, etc. It is important to find out what other clinics are charging. This is called mystery shopping. Ask friends or employees to call all the competitors to find out what they charge per treatment or groups of treatments, who performs it, what system is used, and how long it takes. Ask for informational mailings. Send mystery shoppers in for consultation and treatment to see what is said and done.

Prices per treatment will probably range from $50 or more for an upper lip to $1000 or more for legs. Single treatments or multiple treatment packages may be sold.

In general, for the new laser hair removal clinic, prices should be at the low-to-middle range. The best possible service must be provided,

Do not make it difficult for clients to pay: institute systems to take cash, checks, money orders, and credit cards. Also, do not have clients reconcile accounts over a counter in the waiting area. Create a small, private billing office where the hair removal patients can settle their accounts in a confidential atmosphere. They will always appreciate this.

# Presentation

The presentation of the laser hair removal product will be critical to the success of the clinic's profitability. Presentation links physician, staff, place, price, and even promotion into one harmonious symphony that is known as internal marketing or 'invertising'. Invertising is the summation of all the experiences of the hair removal client, from the time of responding to a promotion to the last treatment. From the time of the first phone call, every single client contact point should be broken down into all the possible events. Physician and staff must script, practice, and orchestrate in such a manner that the experiences or 'through-put' of the clients, as they flow through the clinic, creates a positive experience and encourages them on to the next phase. The summation of all these small co-ordinated bursts of activity is the quality performance of a team that can be successful.

The standard contact phases that must be co-ordinated in the 'through-put' are as follows:

Promotion→Inquiry→Consult→Treatment→Word of mouth→Retreatment→New procedure

The obvious goal is maximizing the client conversion from one phase on to the next. Conversion rates will determine the success and profitability of the clinic. Excellent promotion will generate a large number of leads and consultations. This, through excellent 'invertising', will result in increased treatments. The quality of the product and treatment delivery will maximize word-of-mouth referrals, retreatments and conversions to new procedures.

# Inquiry (Lead Stage)

Promotion (advertising), although technically the first stage of the process, will be covered later. Making the 'phone ring' is usually the easy part. Anyone can utilize funds for adverts that lead to a ringing phone. Where most physicians fail is in maximizing the conversion of phone calls into treatments and retreatments. Unless one prepares for this, a maximum return on advertising or promotional investments will never be achieved.

Each promotional advertising that leads to a call into a hair removal practice will probably cost between $75 and $250 per call, depending upon the advert, the medium and the market. Each time the phone rings, the clinic will either convert that $75–250 call into potential revenue or lost money.

For maximum lead conversion, careful telemarketing scripts must be created. These scripts are the exact responses a physician wants the staff to provide during an introductory phone call. It is this interaction that leads to booking consults. Keep these scripts short, answering common questions, but always emphasizing the benefits of the laser hair removal product. Staff must be focused on the 'closure to consultation' where 'everything will be explained fully'. The script should focus on the unique and positive points of the clinic and its hair removal treatments, including competitive prices and good service. Avoid giving too much information over the phone. Unfortunately, the risk of providing too much information over the phone will increase, as staff become more knowledgeable. Surprisingly, the increased knowledge only increases the risk of staff saying something inaccurate. This can dissuade prospective leads before they can experience the hair removal center's services.

The topic of telemarketing could fill a book itself. There are many books and 1-day courses on this very topic. Success will be documented by measuring conversion rates. Scripts, price, or presentations may occasionally have to be changed. Once the laser clinic is up and running, one should not settle for anything less than a 50% conversion rate of all calls in to consultation. In the beginning, the lead conversions will probably be at a rate of 20–25%. But pay attention to the details of the 10 Ps; individualize the approach to maximize profits. Active leads are the calls that book consultations. Passive leads are the leads that everyone forgets about. These are the callers who did not book a consultation, but have only requested information. Unfortunately, the clinic has already paid for the passive lead phone call ($75–250). These callers must become part of a pool the hair removal clinic continues to access. Part of the telemarketing database will gather necessary demographic data. Consider the mailing of a complimentary information package. The information package is sent to active (consultation booked) and passive (only information requested) leads. It describes the procedure of interest, the physician, the facility, and other services offered. Passive lead management involves a succession of triggered mailings over the first month designed to keep the passive lead (prospective client) interested in the facility. If no consultation is booked after 1 month, the passive lead receives a quarterly newsletter for 2 years. If the passive lead has spent no money in the clinic after 2 years, the prospective client is dropped from the mailing list.

Clearly this kind of lead management or 'contact management' requires the help of a computer software program. These 'contact managers' are abundant. Goldmine™ and ACT™ are a couple of the popular general business contact management programs. Several programs are adapted to the medical practice, such as Nextech™ and Inform and Enhance™. No one program is perfect, but they should offer contact management, triggered mailouts, full reporting, scheduling, and some limited charting. It is difficult to be maximally efficient without one.

# Consultation Phase

As mentioned, the laser hair removal consultation is part encouragement (or 'sales') and part informed consent. The informed consent must be implemented fully, accurately, and ethically. This is even more important in those areas where the cosmetic laser services (including consultation) legally may be delegated to a nurse or technician. The consultation must be broken down into its sales components. A typical hair removal consultation is scheduled for 1 hour. This includes the waiting room 5 minute cross-marketing absorption phase, 30 minutes for the consultation and consent signing, 10 minutes for a possible test spot and assessment, and finally 15 minutes for patient clean-up, make-over, rebooking, account payments, and departure. A staff member who is goal oriented and friendly should assist the patient with all phases.

The consultation is broken into the following elements:

(1) **Be positive**. The goal at the end of a 30-minute consultation is to raise the patient's interest to the point where they will make a booking on the spot. During these concentrated consultation periods, the delegated consultation team (usually the receptionist, physician or nurse, and office manager) must present a positive attitude. Remember much has been spent on (1) the purchase of the lead (promotion), (2) the conversion of that lead into a consultation (telemarketing), and (3) the creation of the right ambiance, atmosphere, marketing literature, and flow through your clinic (presentation). Consultation conversion rates are another stage the clinic will have to live by. It is mandatory that the hair removal clinic projects an organized, confident, well-groomed image.

(2) **Demonstrate your interest in the patient**. For the first 10 minutes of every interview, find out about the patient. It needn't be the physician who does this. Ask about their families, what they enjoy about their work, etc. Try to make a connection that allows the patient to know that you know how interesting they are.

(3) **Find out what the patient really wants**. Ask patients directly what it is they really wish to achieve from hair removal. By getting them to state their goals clearly, the clinic will better be able to service their needs.

(4) **Reassure the patient that you can deliver what they want**. Make sure that laser hair removal can satisfy the specific expectations of the client. The client may have to modify expectations if they are unrealistic (the usual unrealistic patient expectation is 100% permanent hair reduction after one or two treatments).

(5) **Assume the sale**. Carefully word all discussions to include an assumption of purchase of the product. 'Mrs X when you are undergoing your laser hair removal you will find . . .'. Assuming the sale reinforces the urge/impulse of the client to purchase the product. This will translate into a patient undergoing treatment.

(6) **Prevent 'buyer's remorse' (future pacing)**. The patient's mind must be put at ease over expense. This is required to prevent the inevitable remorse experienced by many consumers after a sizable purchase. Patients should be told of the direct benefits of the treatment. As an example, one might ask 'do you have any upcoming social events where the sheer nylons you can purchase after laser hair

removal, will look great?', or 'the vacation you have planned will be so much more enjoyable without having to shave your legs or underarms'.

(7) **The 'closer'.** The 'closer' should always be someone other than the physician, – usually the office manager. This removes the doctor or nurse from discussing finances and squarely keeps them in the role of esthetic health service delivery. The closer is often an individual with sales experience who will be able to convert a higher percentage of consultations to treatments. The closer will also discuss payment terms and options.

Similar to the lead conversion rate, the percentage of consultations leading to laser hair removal treatment should be no less than 50%. In practices with a high percentage of word-of-mouth referrals (clients who come from other happy clients), the closure rate can approach 80–90%. These successful practices are servicing 'buyers'. Buyers are those who call and come knowing they will have treatment. This type of 'buyers' practice is the ideal practice profile, but is usually achieved by 'purchasing' enough 'shoppers' (through promotion) and converting a high percentage of them to happy patients. With attention to the 10 Ps of cosmetic medical marketing, one can achieve this type of practice much sooner. Such a clinic's 'through-put' and service will be superior to its competitors.

For the new laser hair removal clinic, where an exclusive 'buyers practice' does not exist, most clients are simply 'shoppers'. These are patients who were purchased through promotion. 'Shopper practices' need to work very hard with lead and consult conversion to achieve maximum profitability. Most shoppers' practices that attend to service and the 10 Ps should convert at least 50% of consults to treatments.

# Treatment

Like the other stages of contact and conversions, careful consideration must be given to what occurs during the treatment. First and foremost is obvious – treatments must be safe and effective. If the laser hair removal act is delegated to laser nurses or technicians, ensure that they have been well trained. They must know all clinical parameters necessary to safely, autonomously, and effectively deliver the treatment. Create a written 'Delegatable Laser Hair Removal Protocol Document' that clearly outlines the training, continuing education, treatment parameter, and adverse outcome protocol. This document should be kept on file in the clinic, be posted in the laser rooms, and be constantly reviewed and updated. Only when safety and efficacy have been addressed can one focus on presentation, comfort, and promotion.

The laser treatment room should be well decorated, clean, well ventilated and at a comfortable temperature. Provide a comfortable clinic gown, room, slippers, towel(s), and treatment bed. Educate the laser nurse(s) and/or technicians on the other procedures, services, and products provided by the cosmetic clinic. Give them the cross-marketing scripts, skills, and bonus remuneration to allow and motivate them to promote the available services. Ensure that posters, wall-prompts, brochures, and continuously running videos on the other clinic services are exposed or provided to hair removal clients during treatment. Finally, provide a private clinic space for the client to undress, re-apply make-up and freshen up after the treatment before leaving the clinic.

## Word of Mouth, Retreatment, and New Procedure

With a well-delivered laser hair removal product, the majority (over 80%) of patients should return for their 'mandatory' second treatment and over 60–70% should come back two to eight times for retreatments over several years. Retreatment conversion is not only built on the excellent experiences at earlier contact phases, but also depends heavily on the comfortable delivery of the product and its success. Remember: if patients expect 'some' degree of permanent hair reduction and ongoing, intermittent laser hair maintenance at affordable prices, most will be happy to return. A successful hair removal clinic should keep growing; the client base should keep expanding. They will choose other new procedures as well.

One contented hair removal patient can generate an average of four word-of-mouth referrals (and the clinic only paid for the first lead). It is worth sending paying hair removal clients birthday notices and holiday greetings acknowledging your appreciation of their business and perhaps a time-limited discount coupon that can be applied towards clinic services, for each known referral they send. Actively solicit word-of-mouth referrals with mailings to patients and gifts or bonuses (in the form of treatments) if they refer someone.

Conversion is the key to a successful practice. Attention to the 10 Ps will maximize the ability to measure, improve, and control conversion.

## Promotion

Thus far, this chapter has focused on the details of the 'through-put' and the internal marketing details. The surest way to waste money is to promote a practice and product before working out the intricate details of its delivery. If one does not take time with the first few Ps, then one is likely to waste tens of thousands of dollars on advertising with unacceptably low conversion rates.

Promotion can be divided into internal and external promotion. Promotion can be an isolated campaign, usually 6–12 weeks in duration, with one or more media (e.g. radio, newspaper, and direct mail). The advantage of one focused, time-limited promotional campaign is that it saturates the target market for a brief period of time.

---

**Promotion**

*Internal Promotion 'Invertising'*
1. Direct mail – to your existing database
2. Cross-marketing

*External Promotion*
1. Public relations, talks, seminars
2. Public relations consultant/publicist
3. Advertising
   a  Direct mail to targeted postal codes/preferred lists
   b  Internet
   c  Telephone directories (yellow pages)
   d  Radio
   e  Television
   f  Print media, newspapers, magazines

---

Consistent promotion or advert placement is often used on a weekly or bimonthly basis to maintain leads using the best performing medium. Adverts may be strongly 'image oriented' *or* 'call to action' or a combination of 'imaging' *and* 'call to action'. *Image advertising* is easily recognized as the most common form seen on television, radio, and magazines. Image adverts are often run by large companies with a large advertising budget. These are directed to the creation and implementation of ad slicks with an 'image' oriented design. Such an approach allows the consumer to identify with the image; the image becomes brand recognition. Image marketing is not designed for, nor does it require of the consumer, any immediate action. An advert designed to prompt the consumer to pick up the phone and impulsively/decisively call a number is called *call to action* advertising.

Cosmetic laser surgery adverts are often examples of a combined 'image' and 'call to action'. Because laser aesthetic services are a very visual product, imagery evokes strong emotion and consumer impulses. A laser hair removal advert showing before and after images of a model's long smooth legs would be such an example. However, most medical practices cannot afford to place image adverts with the hope that patients will call for a consultation. Medical practices are not usually large corporations. A medical practice must produce immediate leads and business with its advertising dollars. A medical practice may entice the patient with image marketing. This must be followed by a strong 'call to action' such as 'call now for a free consultation' or 'upper lip hair removal at a $99 discount for the first 100 callers'. In medical advertising combinations of strong imagery, bold print, before and afters, strong calls to action, and the word 'free' usually generate an adequate number of leads with low 'lead costs'.

'**Lead cost**' is the amount it costs to acquire each phone call (lead) resulting from a specific advert. The calculation is very easy. It is an automatic component of most reports in contact management systems. It is the cost of the specific advert divided by the number of leads attributed to that advert. For example, if an advert costs $3000 to implement and generates 30 calls over the next 3–4 weeks, the lead cost is $3000/30 = $100. As a rule, in laser hair removal where the product price per treatment may average only $500, the lead cost cannot exceed more than $100 per call.

# Internal Marketing 'Invertising'

### Direct Mail

For practices with large existing patient bases, direct mail is where promotion should begin. Primary practitioners, internists, and dermatologists often have large rosters of long-term repeat patients. These patients already know and trust their physicians. These physicians might be said to have 'brand recognition'. The lead conversion rates should approach 80% (converting leads to consults) and should be around $20–50/lead. Here the cost is a simple direct mail campaign to existing patients. The group most interested is female patients of 20–65 years of age. A mass mailing to existing patients, describing the new laser hair removal services, should cost $2000 for 5000 mailouts. This simple campaign should generate 40–50 calls ($50 lead cost).

This routine can give the physician and staff a trial run of both the presentation and 'through-put' the clinic has developed with the most accessible group of clients. This simple example can improve the telemarketing, consultation, and treatment skills on existing, satisfied patients. This should always be the first trial before the clinic goes out and 'buys shoppers' through more expensive promotion activities.

### Cross-Marketing

All patients who come to the office should receive the 'clinic awareness' materials (customized brochures, videos on show, posters) of all available services. Remember to track the cost of these materials and the percentages of patients who come from these activities. These lead to an assessment of efficacy and possibly alterations of the approach.

# External Marketing

This comprises all promotional activities that reach outside the existing practice. The lead costs below are given as a guide. One should utilize the advertising departments of newspapers and magazines or employ the services of an advertising agency ($2000–$3000 per advert). It is worth trying different media, but above all, the efficacy of the method should be measured. If an advert does not work, and enough calls are not generated, lead costs will be too high. Anything above $150 is too high for laser hair removal. By measuring lead costs, promotions can be adjusted. If the advert does not work, then the wrong medium may have been chosen (try another) or the message may be poorly designed (change it). Do not be satisfied until lead costs are $125/lead or lower.

## Public Relations

Make an effort to speak at various medical societies and women's groups that match the target market. Given the expense of a physician's time, the lead cost of these activities will be very high. However, this is a good way to generate awareness during the start-up phase of a hair removal clinic.

## Public Relations Consultant

If laser activities and services are the only offered services, then the lead costs of $200–500 for a consultant will be too expensive. However, a good public relations consultant can be indispensible to a large multiservice practice in the long run. especially if other cosmetic surgical procedures are offered. A good public relations consultant will generate awareness and media stories about the physician, the clinic, and its services. It doesn't take long to become known as a laser esthetic expert.

## Internet

One-time start-up costs of $1000–6000 and maintenance of $500/year are quite expensive. Initial lead costs, due to the one-time start-up expense, may prohibit this. But lead costs decrease with time (due to the one-time nature of the expense). A web site also serves as an information center somewhat akin to the yellow pages, for people who use the Internet. However, it is worth noting that a high proportion of women aged 20–65 do not, as yet, use the Internet. It is estimated that the percentage of female Internet users will increase by at least 100% per year for the next 10 years. So it is wise to consider going 'on line'. However, do not expect that a web site will keep the hair removal clinic busy in the beginning.

## Radio

Effective 30- and 60-second spots on the radio usually cannot be achieved with lead costs of less than $150. Such costs usually make this medium too expensive.

## Television

Lead costs of $175–250 are again too expensive for hair removal (remember, the average treatment expenditure is $500).

### Direct Mail

Such lists are purchased from a variety of companies. These are like direct 'cold calls' with lead costs of $200 or more for laser hair removal alone. Success rates are not high.

### Telephone Directories

Telephone directory ('yellow page') advertisements are indispensable. They generate leads themselves, as well as supporting leads generated from other promotional activities. When measured by themselves yellow pages' lead costs of $150–200 can be expected. However, because leads generated from other promotional media such as newspapers, radio, etc., often look for the clinic number in the yellow pages, their supportive and integrated value cannot be ignored. It is not worth purchasing full-page, four-color adverts in multiple telephone books. Unless the laser hair clinic has other more expensive cosmetic services to offer, the fees of up to $10,000/month are not worthwhile.

### Magazines

Line rates in magazines are more expensive than similar rates in newspapers. However the adverts are more attractive and their 'shelf life' is longer. Conversely, the market reach is usually smaller with magazine adverts. In general, lead costs of $150 can be achieved with magazine-generated adverts.

### Newspapers

As a general rule, the newspaper generates the lowest lead costs for laser hair removal. If there is more than one daily newspaper in the target area, research which newspaper reaches the greatest percentage of your likely patients (women 20–65 and making over $30,000). A large launch advert with a subsequent weekly presence preceding and during peak hair removal times (fall, winter, spring) should result in lead costs between $75 and $235. These adverts should be a combination of image advertising, with a story about the product, and a strong 'call to action'.

# PRECISION AND PREDICTABILITY

Conversion rates will determine a clinic's success and profitability. Implementing the 10 Ps will help maximize conversions. Measurements of conversions must always be made. Measurements lead to adjustments, re-engineering and alterations of the process at each contact stage. Remember:

Advert → Lead → Consultation → Treatment → Retreatment → Word-of-mouth

By measuring, one knows the precise conversion rates for each stage. Any time the conversion rate falls below optimum standards, adjustments become mandatory. If the clinic is already converting at 50%, do not accept this. Strive for 75 or 90%.

Measure conversions weekly. Staff bonuses should be based on optimal rates. By conducting weekly staff meetings where conversion rates are discussed, sudden drops in otherwise optimal rates will often reveal a cause. There might be an inadvertent change in protocol or a staff interpersonal and/or family crisis. Measurement will be the key to micromanagement of a successful laser hair removal practice. Measurement will give one the power to control practice flow and profitability.

The following, then, are the measurements that must be tracked.

(1)  Referral source cost
     (advertising cost)
(2)  Lead cost = Cost of advert/no. of leads (calls)
     – keep less than $125, aim for $75
     – measures success of the advert (or promotion)
(3)  Lead conversion rate = no. of leads/no. of consultations
     – percentage of leads converted to consults
     – measures telemarketing success
     – keep over 50%, aim for >75%
(4)  Consult conversion rate = no. of treatments/no. of consultations
     – measures success of consultation phase
     – keep over 50%, aim for 75%
(5)  Retreatment conversion = no. of retreatments/no. of treatments
     – percentage of clients who return for retreatment
     – measures success of the treatment phase
     – keep over 75% between hair removal treatment 1 and 2 and 50% thereafter
(6)  Word-of-mouth referral rate = no. of word of mouth referrals/no. of treatments
     – percentage of patients who refer other patients
     – aim for 25%
(7)  Return on Investment (ROI) = revenue in sales from an advert/cost of the advert
     – return on investment for each advertising dollar
     – minimal acceptable ROI should be 3:1, that is $3 in revenue for each dollar of advertising
     – aim for 10:1 to 15:1 with retreatment and word-of-mouth referrals augmenting the profitability from the initial lead costs

# PROFITABILITY AND PLEASURE

By using the 10 Ps as a template to construct a laser hair removal practice, happy patients will be the result. These clients, in turn, generate word-of-mouth referrals, which make for a successful program. With this profitability, and self-determination, comes pleasure. It is this pleasure that leads to enjoyment. A laser hair removal practice can be lucrative, stimulating, and pleasurable.

# INDEX